EXCLUDING FRAUDULENT PROVIDERS FROM MEDICAID

HEARING

BEFORE THE

SUBCOMMITTEE ON HUMAN RESOURCES AND INTERGOVERNMENTAL RELATIONS

OF THE

COMMITTEE ON GOVERNMENT REFORM AND OVERSIGHT
HOUSE OF REPRESENTATIVES

ONE HUNDRED FOURTH CONGRESS

SECOND SESSION

SEPTEMBER 5, 1996

Printed for the use of the Committee on Government Reform and Oversight

U.S. GOVERNMENT PRINTING OFFICE

44–731   WASHINGTON : 1997

For sale by the U.S. Government Printing Office
Superintendent of Documents, Congressional Sales Office, Washington, DC 20402
ISBN 0-16-055925-1

CONTENTS

EXCLUDING FRAUDULENT PROVIDERS FROM MEDICAID

THURSDAY, SEPTEMBER 5, 1996

House of Representatives,
Subcommittee on Human Resources and
Intergovernmental Relations,
Committee on Government Reform and Oversight,
Washington, DC.

The subcommittee met, pursuant to notice, at 10:20 a.m., in room 2247, Rayburn House Office Building, Hon. Christopher Shays (chairman of the subcommittee) presiding.

Present: Representatives Shays, Schiff, Souder, Towns and Green.

Staff present: Lawrence J. Halloran, staff director and counsel; Robert Newman, professional staff member; Thomas M. Costa, clerk; and Cheryl Phelps, minority professional staff member.

Mr. SHAYS. I want to apologize to the Members. I was at the Rules Committee. I should have called the committee and let them start without me, and I apologize for not doing that, and I apologize to the witnesses as well.

I call this hearing to order.

When it takes months or years to exclude fraudulent and abusive providers from Medicaid, sick people are endangered, and the physical integrity of their health care is undermined. When providers excluded from one State's Medicaid program slip past our defenses and continue to drain resources from Medicare, that program, too, is put at risk.

In this hearing, we ask why the current system to bar providers from Medicaid is so cumbersome, paper intensive, and prone to error, and what can be done do make the exclusion sanction more effective?

At this subcommittee's request, the General Accounting Office, [GAO] undertook an indepth examination of the Medicaid provider exclusion process in four States and the District of Columbia. Their findings point to a national system plagued by lengthy delays, inconsistent standards, and a serious lack of information-sharing and coordination.

As a result, the GAO finds providers considered unfit to participate in one State's Medicaid program can continue to bill other States' programs as well as Medicare.

This happens because provider fraud and patient abuse are ubiquitous, while the exclusion sanction is prodding and rare. In an age of computerized recordkeeping, when the States and the Health Care Financing Administration [HCFA] boast about their ability to

(1)

pay claims at the speed of light, the policing of those to whom we pay those claims seems to grope along by candlelight.

It is a complex, labor-intense, paper-based system which eventually adds names to the national exclusion list. The GAO found it can take anywhere from a month to a year or more just to assemble the paperwork needed to impose a national exclusion. While the inspector general [IG], and the State agency exchange phone calls, send letters, and retrieve documents, a provider already convicted of health care fraud or patient abuse can continue to bill other Federal health programs.

In this process, State Medicaid fraud control units, Medicaid agencies, and State professional licensing boards all make determinations affecting a provider's right to participate in Medicaid. That is as it should be. Medicaid is an intergovernmental partnership, and the States play an indispensable role in protecting the program's operational and financial integrity.

Our State witnesses today will describe their work as the first line of defense against fraudulent Medicaid providers.

At the national level, the HHS inspector general must gather the results of 54 separate State and territorial administrative or court proceedings and decide whether those actions meet the Federal statutory criteria for mandatory or permissive exclusion from Medicaid, Medicare and other Federal procurements. Only then is a provider added to the sanction list, only then.

Health care payers seeking to find out whether a doctor, nurse, pharmacist, or even a cab driver is on the list must undertake a manual search, and hope enough information matches to allow identification of an excluded provider.

Obviously, so cumbersome a system can be evaded by unscrupulous providers who can change addresses or take on a new corporate form while continuing to abuse patients and defraud public funds. So complex and labor intensive a process also strains already scarce enforcement resources.

Since our hearing on this topic last year, the inspector general has made some improvements to the management of the exclusion system. The cumulative sanction list is now available on the Internet, as are the monthly additions also published in the *Federal Register*. But the IG and the GAO agree that more can be done, must be done to improve the consistency and effectiveness of Medicaid provider exclusions. We will hear their suggestions today.

Finally, I note with some satisfaction that provisions of the recently enacted Health Care Portability and Accountability Act, the health care reform bill, strengthen the exclusion sanction. Those provisions, first offered in legislation sponsored by Mr. Schiff and myself last year as well as our ranking member, expand mandatory exclusion criteria to include conviction of felony health care fraud, the new Federal criminal offense that, for the first time, protects all health care payers, both public and private.

The health care reform law also sets minimum periods for certain permissive exclusions and makes additional resources available for these enforcement activities.

Consistent with the legislation considered by this subcommittee, the new law also directs the HHS Secretary to move toward implementation of a system of unique identification or billing numbers for health care providers. We asked HCFA to describe today their work in this area and help assess how and when such a system might make identification of excluded providers easier and more reliable.

The success of the strengthened sanctions depends on concerted, timely efforts by the IG, HCFA and the States, and we seek your comments today on how those reforms will be implemented.

Again, we welcome all witnesses here today, and we look forward to their testimony.

And again, I would like to apologize for being late. Mr. Towns.

Mr. TOWNS. Thank you very much, Mr. Chairman. First of all, I would like to commend you on holding this hearing. I think it's a very important hearing because we're talking about saving dollars.

Last year, Medicaid accounted for $156 billion in total spending, of which the Federal portion was $89 billion. It is estimated that more than $15 billion in State and Federal Medicaid funds was lost to fraudulent and abusive practices in fiscal year 1995.

Mr. Chairman, controlling the fiscal hemorrhage can recapture potentially billions of taxpayers' dollars. Also, as the recently signed welfare reform legislation will require shifting Medicaid completely to State control, the need for effective, uniform anti-fraud procedures has never been more acute.

This is the ninth hearing this subcommittee has convened to examine health care fraud and abuse. Among the facts we have established is that fraudulent and substandard providers can migrate in and out of the health care system unless provisions are in place to effectively and consistently exclude them.

The Social Security Act provides the inspector general a wide range of mandatory and permissive authorities to exclude providers from federally sponsored health programs; and three additional exclusion provisions were added with the passage of the Kennedy-Kassebaum bill.

However, it is the responsibility of the States to first identify and sanction fraudulent providers within their own programs and also make use of exclusion notices to bar sanctioned providers from their programs.

More than 8,800 Medicaid providers are actively excluded from the Federal health program. This is the number since 1977.

In fiscal year 1995, 1,247 exclusion actions were imposed. Nevertheless, serious questions have been raised that Medicaid excluded providers often continue to profit from the Federal health programs due to a number of systemic deficiencies at the State as well as at the Federal level.

Mr. Chairman, I look forward to the testimony of today's witnesses so that we might clarify exactly what the obstacles are to excluding fraudulent and substandard providers from Federal health programs.

In addition, I look forward to working with you, the administration, the States and others to identify opportunities to correct these problems.

So with that in mind, Mr. Chairman, I yield back the balance of my time, and I accept your apology for being late.

[The prepared statement of Hon. Edolphus Towns follows:]

OPENING STATEMENT OF
THE HON. EDOLPHUS TOWNS
COMMITTEE ON GOVERNMENT REFORM AND OVERSIGHT

"EXCLUDING FRAUDULENT PROVIDERS FROM MEDICAID"

September 5, 1996

LAST YEAR, MEDICAID ACCOUNTED FOR $156 BILLION IN TOTAL SPENDING, OF WHICH THE FEDERAL PORTION WAS $89 BILLION. IT IS ESTIMATED THAT MORE THAT $15 BILLION IN STATE AND FEDERAL MEDICAID FUNDS WAS LOST TO FRAUDULENT AND ABUSIVE PRACTICES IN FISCAL YEAR 1995.

MR. CHAIRMAN, CONTROLLING THIS FISCAL HEMORRHAGE CAN RECAPTURE POTENTIALLY BILLIONS OF TAXPAYER DOLLARS. ALSO, AS THE RECENTLY SIGNED WELFARE REFORM LEGISLATION WILL REQUIRE SHIFTING MEDICAID COMPLETELY TO STATE CONTROL -- THE NEED FOR EFFECTIVE, UNIFORM ANTI-FRAUD PROCEDURES HAS NEVER BEEN MORE ACUTE.

THIS IS THE NINTH HEARING THE SUBCOMMITTEE HAS CONVENED TO EXAMINE HEALTH CARE FRAUD AND ABUSE. AMONG THE FACTS WE HAVE ESTABLISHED IS THAT FRAUDULENT AND SUBSTANDARD PROVIDERS CAN MIGRATE IN AND OUT OF THE HEALTH CARE SYSTEM UNLESS PROVISIONS ARE IN PLACE TO EFFECTIVELY AND CONSISTENTLY EXCLUDE THEM.

THE SOCIAL SECURITY ACT PROVIDES THE INSPECTOR GENERAL A WIDE RANGE OF MANDATORY AND PERMISSIVE AUTHORITIES TO EXCLUDE PROVIDERS FROM FEDERALLY-SPONSORED HEALTH PROGRAMS; AND THREE ADDITIONAL EXCLUSION PROVISIONS WERE ADDED WITH THE PASSAGE OF THE KENNEDY-KASSEBAUM HEALTH INSURANCE LEGISLATION. HOWEVER, IT IS THE RESPONSIBILITY OF THE STATES TO FIRST IDENTIFY AND SANCTION FRAUDULENT PROVIDERS WITHIN THEIR OWN PROGRAMS -- AND ALSO MAKE USE OF THE EXCLUSION NOTICES TO BAR SANCTIONED PROVIDERS FROM THEIR PROGRAMS.

MORE THAN 8800 MEDICAID PROVIDERS ARE ACTIVELY EXCLUDED FROM FEDERAL HEALTH PROGRAMS. IN FISCAL YEAR 1995, 1247 EXCLUSION ACTIONS WERE IMPOSED. NEVERTHELESS, SERIOUS QUESTIONS HAVE BEEN RAISED THAT MEDICAID-EXCLUDED PROVIDERS OFTEN CONTINUE TO PROFIT FROM FEDERAL HEALTH PROGRAMS DUE TO A NUMBER OF SYSTEMIC DEFICIENCIES AT THE STATE AS WELL AS THE FEDERAL LEVEL.

ONE OBSTACLE TO EFFECTIVE NATIONWIDE EXCLUSION SANCTIONS THAT HAS OFTEN BEEN CITED IS THE ORGANIZATIONAL, RESOURCE, AND PROCEDURAL INCONSISTENCIES AMONG THE 50 STATES AND THE FEDERAL GOVERNMENT. ANOTHER IS THE UTILITY OF DATA PROVIDED TO STATES ON EXCLUSION CASES. ANOTHER IS THE FAILURE OF SOME STATES TO USE THE LIST OF EXCLUDED PROVIDERS APPROPRIATELY. A FOURTH IS THE DELAY IN DECISION-MAKING IN THE OFFICE OF THE INSPECTOR GENERAL.

MR. CHAIRMAN, I LOOK FORWARD TO THE TESTIMONY OF TODAY'S WITNESSES SO THAT WE MIGHT CLARIFY EXACTLY WHAT THE OBSTACLES ARE TO EXCLUDING FRAUDULENT AND SUBSTANDARD PROVIDERS FROM FEDERAL HEALTH PROGRAMS.   IN ADDITION, I LOOK FORWARD TO WORKING WITH YOU, THE ADMINISTRATION, THE STATES, AND OTHERS TO IDENTIFY OPPORTUNITIES TO CORRECT THESE OBSTACLES.

Mr. SHAYS. Thank you. No. I do appreciate that. It's not my practice to be late. Before calling on our two distinguished Members, I would like to ask unanimous consent that all members of the subcommittee be permitted to place any opening statements in the record and that the record remain open for 3 days for that purpose. Without objection, so ordered.

And I also ask unanimous consent that our witnesses be permitted to include their written testimony in the record. Without objection, so ordered.

At this time I would acknowledge that Rufus Noble, the inspector general from the Health Care Administration staff of Florida, will not be here due to the Hurricane Fran in Florida.

We'll miss his testimony.

At this time I call on our very active Member and very effective Member, the vice chairman of the subcommittee, Mr. Souder.

Mr. SOUDER. Thank you for that, but I don't have any comment.

Mr. SHAYS. OK. Mr. Schiff, my colleague-in-arms here.

Mr. SCHIFF. Mr. Chairman, I think you, and our ranking member said it all.

Mr. SHAYS. OK.

Mr. SCHIFF. And I'm glad to have worked with you on legislation in this area and know there is a lot more to do and look forward to working with you again on this. Thank you.

Mr. SHAYS. Thank you, Mr. Schiff. I just want to point out to our witnesses in the audience that this committee takes tremendous pride and interest in these hearings.

Our hearings last year generated making health care fraud an all-payer fraud in the health care reform bill. So these aren't just hearings. These are hearings that result in meaningful legislation, and we treat it very seriously and know that you do as well.

But we learn a lot from the hearings, and ultimately, you see the results of the hearings in legislation.

With that, I will call our first witness, Leslie Aronovitz, who is the Associate Director of Health Financing and Public Health, General Accounting Office, accompanied by Katherine Allen, Assistant Director, Health Financing Issues; and Robert Ferschl, senior evaluator, as well.

Now, I should have asked you to remain standing, because we swear in all our witnesses.

[Witnesses sworn.]

Mr. SHAYS. For the record, all three of our witnesses have responded in the affirmative, and we invite you to have your testimony. Will all three of you be giving testimony?

Ms. ARONOVITZ. No. I'll just be giving testimony.

Mr. SHAYS. But all three will respond to our questions?

Ms. ARONOVITZ. They're very knowledgeable about a lot of the issues you might bring up.

Mr. SHAYS. Thank you for bringing them. OK.

STATEMENT OF LESLIE ARONOVITZ, ASSOCIATE DIRECTOR, HEALTH FINANCING AND PUBLIC HEALTH, GENERAL ACCOUNTING OFFICE, ACCOMPANIED BY KATHRYN ALLEN, ASSISTANT DIRECTOR, HEALTH FINANCING ISSUES; AND ROBERT FERSCHL, SENIOR EVALUATOR

Ms. ARONOVITZ. Mr. Chairman, and members of the subcommittee, I am pleased to be here today to discuss our ongoing work related to excluded health care providers.

I would like to introduce my colleagues one more time. On my right is Kathy Allen, who is an Assistant Director in our Health Financing group in Washington. And on my left is Bob Ferschl, who works on health issues out of our Chicago field office.

We focused our work on health care providers who have been removed from their State Medicaid programs for committing fraud or rendering substandard care to beneficiaries. When this occurs, the HHS–OIG is responsible for determining whether such circumstances warrant prompt exclusion nationwide from all Federal health programs. Our work responds to your concern that despite the OIG's efforts, providers who have been convicted of fraud and who have delivered inadequate or inappropriate care may still be participating in these programs.

We performed our work in six States and four OIG field offices. I now learn that two of them have been combined. As of September 3, it was the Philadelphia and Washington, DC, offices. And we met with OIG officials at headquarters.

Although the OIG has excluded thousands of providers, our work suggests that several weaknesses in its process can leave many other sanctioned providers on the rolls of Federal health programs for unacceptable periods of time. I'd like to briefly discuss some of these weaknesses.

The first has to do with lengthy delays in the OIG's decision process. In reviewing the OIG's exclusion of State-referred cases, we identified a number of cases, including those involving mandatory exclusions or serious quality of care issues that remained unresolved for long periods of time with no apparent explanation for the delays. In one case, for example, a pharmacy was terminated for overbilling the Illinois Medicaid Program by over $117,000. It took the Chicago field office 15 months to forward the case to headquarters for exclusion. The case file showed no activity for extended periods of time, including a 10-month period.

Another weakness we identified in the OIG's process involves inconsistencies among its field offices and how they use their discretionary authority and the types of cases they refer to headquarters. This is especially true for permissive cases where there is a lot of discretion on the part of the IG as to what cases will be considered for exclusion nationwide. As a result, providers with equally serious problems could be treated differently by the OIG, depending on their location.

We attempted to identify the magnitude of problems we found in the exclusion process, but we were unable to do so primarily because of a lack of case file documentation at the field offices. For example, the Chicago field office could not locate 5 of 17 referrals sent by a State Medicaid agency during 1994 and 1995. As a result, it could not confirm that it had received the referrals or explain why it had not considered exclusion. Our review of these five cases at the State Medicaid agency determined that three of them involved serious quality of care issues.

I'd like to briefly turn now to some issues we identified at the State level that relate to their referral patterns and their response to the OIG's exclusion list.

During our State visits, we found that, in some circumstances, Illinois permits providers to voluntarily withdraw from its Medicaid Program.

And also, in New York, they terminate their Medicaid contract, rather than subject these providers to formal sanction, in some circumstances.

These actions quickly remove aberrant providers or potentially aberrant providers from State Medicaid programs. However, these cases are not reported to the OIG even though some of them appear to be serious quality of care problems.

For example, a podiatrist withdrew voluntarily. We say voluntarily in quotes because we don't believe he would have stood up and volunteered unless he felt that there was severe evidence against him in terms of his ability to deliver quality care. But he withdrew from the Illinois program in August 1995, after the State alleged that he had provided grossly inferior care to Medicaid recipients.

But because he was never referred to the OIG, he continued to participate in Medicare and has received over $20,000 providing services to program beneficiaries.

So even though he can't treat my children, he could probably treat my mother in Medicare, although she doesn't live in Illinois.

While Illinois and New York's aggressive action results in safeguards for those State's Medicaid programs, it affords no protection from Medicare and other State's Medicaid programs.

We do not know how prevalent voluntary withdrawals are nationwide. The other four States we went to told us that they did not allow providers to withdraw from their programs and instead waited for a formal sanction from, let's say, a licensing board.

The problem is that if you wait for a licensing board, it's possible that this could severely extend the amount of time that the person is under investigation and has a chance to appeal. And therefore, not only are Medicare and other beneficiaries from other Federal health programs at risk during that time, but also Medicaid recipients are also at risk because they would not be removed from that program immediately. So it is a two-edged sword, but we have some ideas about that.

Finally, I'd like to address States response to the OIG notification process. In addition to the letters sent to the States, when a provider is excluded, the OIG widely disseminates information on excluded providers through monthly reports and periodic cumulative listings to various State and Federal agencies.

We found, however, that for several reasons States sometimes have difficulty identifying and excluding providers who appear on these lists.

First, the States have difficulty identifying individuals such as nurses, pharmacists, or physicians who are employed by hospitals, nursing homes, pharmacies, and health maintenance organizations that bill the program under the entity's billing number and not the provider number itself.

They're called unenrolled providers and they can hide—be employed by one of these other entities—and not be detected.

We also found that providers sometimes are not identified because States tend to use the OIG's monthly list for a one-time check against their active provider files, but they don't flag these providers in case they subsequently apply to the program.

Finally, some States do not always check providers appearing on the OIG list who have out-of-state addresses.

When we performed a computer match of the OIG exclusion list to Illinois' enrolled provider file, we found 13 out-of-state providers who had been excluded by the OIG between 1988 and 1995 but were still enrolled in the Illinois Medicaid Program.

One of them had received almost $25,000 in Medicaid payments since being excluded by the OIG. One other issue that you mentioned in your statement is that of putting the OIG exclusion list on the Internet.

We think that any broad dissemination of this list is very positive. However, any information that's accessed to the public does not include any type of provider identification numbers like Social Security numbers or billing numbers, which makes it much more difficult for States to be able to do computer matches or manipulate the information.

Also, in many States, we found that States give providers an opportunity to use an employer identification number, an EIN, or an SSN.

And in that case, it's also very difficult to assure that you have the right provider when you're doing a match, because you want to make sure that you have the right identifier, and sometimes they're different in different States.

So this creates a lot of challenges for States. Our work to date shows that the opportunity exists for and, indeed, we found many cases where providers deemed to be unfit to participate in one State's Medicaid program can continue to do so in the Medicare Program or Medicaid in other States.

The OIG has several initiatives underway that I'm sure Ms. Brown will describe to you. Also, recent enactment of the Health Insurance Portability and Accountability Act of 1996 will provide additional resources to the OIG that could remedy some of these problems.

However, in the short term, we have been discussing very specific actions that the OIG could take in several areas that would substantially improve its effectiveness.

For example, the OIG could provide more guidance for its field office staff and the States to facilitate prompt preparation of case files, including required documentation that the OIG needs to make its decision.

It could also clarify guidance for the field offices to ensure more consistency in the cases that are sent forward to headquarters for a final decision.

Furthermore, it could explore ways to ensure that States quickly identify and act to remove OIG-excluded providers and listen to some of the problems that the States say they have in terms of the cumbersomeness of the OIG exclusion lists.

Finally, the OIG may want to ask States to begin reporting information on those providers who agree to withdraw from a State Medicaid Program rather than subject themselves to the formal sanction process.

This concludes my formal statement, and I'll be happy to respond to any questions you or any other members of the subcommittee may have.

[The prepared statement of Ms. Aronovitz follows:]

Mr. Chairman and Members of the Subcommittee:

I am pleased to be here today to discuss our ongoing work related to health care providers who have been removed from their state Medicaid programs for committing program fraud or rendering substandard care to beneficiaries. When this occurs, the Department of Health and Human Services' (HHS) Office of the Inspector General (OIG) is responsible for determining whether such circumstances warrant prompt nationwide exclusion of those providers from all federal health programs. Our work responds to your concern that despite the OIG's efforts, providers who have been convicted of fraud or who have delivered inadequate or inappropriate care may still be participating in these programs.

My comments today will focus on the process the OIG uses for excluding providers from Medicaid, Medicare, and other federal health programs. Our objective was to determine whether this process effectively ensures that excluded providers do not continue to participate in these programs.

In developing this information, we visited the District of Columbia, Illinois, Maryland, Missouri, and Virginia. For these five states,[1] we worked with officials of state Medicaid agencies, licensing boards, and Medicare contractors to document their exclusion processes. We performed computer matches of OIG and state lists of excluded providers and Medicare claims data. We also reviewed case files for a judgmentally selected sample of excluded providers to determine the nature of their wrongdoing and the types of sanctions they received. We also performed limited work in New York State to understand the state Medicaid program's exclusion process. In addition, we met with officials from the four OIG field offices--Chicago, New York, Philadelphia, and Washington, D.C.--that oversee these six states, and with OIG headquarters officials.

In brief, although the OIG has excluded thousands of providers, our work suggests that several weaknesses in its process can leave sanctioned providers on the rolls of federal health programs for unacceptable periods of time. This puts at risk the health and safety of beneficiaries and compromises the financial integrity of Medicaid, Medicare, and other federal health programs. The weaknesses we identified include (1) lengthy delays in the OIG's decision process, even in cases where a provider has been convicted of fraud or patient abuse or neglect; (2) inconsistencies among OIG field offices regarding which providers will be considered for nationwide exclusion; (3) states not informing the OIG about providers who agree to stop participating in their Medicaid programs even though the reason for agreeing to withdraw is sometimes egregious patient care or abusive billing; and (4) how

---

[1]For the purposes of this discussion, we include the District of Columbia as a state.

states use information from the OIG to remove excluded providers from state programs.

In addition to identifying these system weaknesses, we attempted to assess the magnitude of these problems. Incomplete records in the OIG field offices where we conducted work did not permit such an analysis, however. We therefore could not identify the universe of cases referred to the OIG field offices, determine if all cases received were reviewed and acted upon in a timely manner, or obtain the rationale for decisions not to recommend exclusion to headquarters.

<u>BACKGROUND</u>

Medicaid is a joint federal-state health program for the poor that expended $159 billion in fiscal year 1995 to provide health care coverage for over 40 million people. Because of its size and complex structure, Medicaid is vulnerable to fraud and abuse. State Medicaid agencies have the primary responsibility to protect the program's financial integrity and to ensure that beneficiaries have access to quality care. This includes ensuring that appropriate safeguards are in place to remove providers that commit fraud or abuse, or are incompetent, from state programs.

At the federal level, the Secretary of HHS has delegated to the OIG the authority under sections 1128 and 1156 of the Social Security Act to exclude health care providers from most federal health care programs.[2] The OIG, through its Office of Investigations, is required to exclude, nationwide, providers who have been convicted of Medicare- or Medicaid-related fraud and patient abuse or neglect, and felonies related to health care fraud and controlled substances.[3] These actions are termed "mandatory exclusions."

---

[2]OIG exclusions are effective with respect to Medicare (title XVIII of the Social Security Act) and state health care programs, defined as Medicaid (title XIX), Maternal and Child Health Services Block grant (title V), and Block Grants to States for Social Services (title XX). As a result of the Federal Acquisition Streamlining Act of 1994, which mandates and expands the governmentwide effect of all debarments, suspensions, and other exclusionary actions to federal procurement and nonprocurement programs, OIG exclusions also apply to health care providers participating in the Federal Employees' Health Benefits Program (FEHBP) administered by the U.S. Office of Personnel Management and the Civilian Health and Medical Program of the Uniformed Services (CHAMPUS) administered by the Department of Defense.

[3]These latter two mandatory exclusions were recently added by the Health Insurance Portability and Accountability Act of 1996.

The OIG also has authority to exclude other individuals or entities if the OIG determines that the particular facts in a case meet its criteria. These so-called "permissive exclusions" may be based on, for example, submitting excessive claims, license suspensions and revocations, and sanctions imposed by federal or state health agencies. (See the appendix for a complete list of exclusion authorities.)

The OIG field offices receive referrals of sanction actions taken by state Medicaid agencies, licensing boards, Medicaid fraud control units (MFCU),[4] and others. For mandatory cases, they assemble and forward to headquarters the case files containing evidence of a provider's criminal conviction. For referrals falling under the permissive exclusion authorities, the field offices receive documents related to disciplinary actions taken by state Medicaid agencies, licensing boards, or others. They assess the relevant facts and forward to OIG headquarters the cases they recommend for exclusion. OIG headquarters makes the final decision about whether to exclude the provider from program participation.

When the OIG excludes a provider, it sends notification letters to organizations such as state Medicaid agencies, Medicare claims-processing contractors, state licensing boards, and MFCUs in the states where the provider is known to practice or operate. When applicable, the provider's employer is also notified. In addition, information on excluded providers is disseminated nationally through monthly reports and semiannual cumulative listings.

As of February 1996--the latest date for which cumulative data were prepared--the OIG had excluded 8,830 providers from federal health care programs nationwide. Three exclusion categories-- conviction for program-related crime, conviction for patient abuse or neglect, and license suspensions and revocations--accounted for 76 percent of these nationwide exclusions.

OIG PROCESS DOES NOT ENSURE THAT ALL PROVIDERS ARE EXCLUDED IN A TIMELY MANNER

In reviewing the OIG's exclusion of state-referred cases, we identified a number of cases--including those involving mandatory exclusions or serious quality of care issues--that remained unresolved for long periods of time. In the Chicago and Washington field offices, for example, we found delays that were due, at least in part, to state Medicaid agencies and MFCUs not always submitting

---

[4]Most states have MFCUs that must be organizationally independent of the agency that operates the state Medicaid program. A MFCU is usually a component of the state attorney general's office. MFCUs investigate and prosecute provider fraud and cases relating to neglect or abuse of patients in nursing homes and other facilities.

documentation the field offices needed to process the exclusion.
Thus, the completeness of the documentation provided by these
agencies varied, necessitating frequent back-and-forth telephone
contacts and correspondence to obtain data. The Washington field
office advised us that it could take as long as 2 months to obtain
needed documentation from state agencies.

In other instances, however, case files showed long periods of
inactivity with no apparent explanation for the delays. In one
case, a pharmacy was terminated for overbilling the Illinois
Medicaid program by over $117,000. It took the Chicago field
office 15 months to forward the case to headquarters for exclusion.
The case file showed no activity for extended periods of time,
including a 10-month period. In another case, the field office
referred a provider to headquarters for exclusion 19 months after
the Illinois MFCU notified it that the provider had pled guilty in
state court to falsely billing for Medicaid services. Two and one-
half months after the case was forwarded to OIG headquarters, the
provider was excluded nationwide.

INCONSISTENCIES AMONG FIELD OFFICES

Another weakness we identified in the OIG's process involves
inconsistencies among its field offices in how they use their
discretionary authority and the types of cases they refer to
headquarters. This is especially true in the case of permissive
exclusions, where the field offices may decide whether to recommend
exclusion.

In 1987, the OIG was given expanded discretionary authority to
exclude providers nationwide.[5] Our work to date, however,
indicates that the OIG has not always used its expanded exclusion
authority as widely as it could. OIG officials told us that given
the OIG's competing priorities, permissive exclusions have
sometimes taken a lower priority. In October 1992, the OIG
instructed its field offices to only process state Medicaid agency
and licensing board disciplinary actions in which there was actual
harm to patients and in which the provider had moved to another
state. Field offices asked state agencies to only report these
types of cases. About 1 year later, however, the OIG rescinded
this guidance and state agencies were asked to once again refer all
cases.

We also observed apparent inconsistencies in the way field
offices are processing permissive cases. As a result, providers
with equally serious problems could be treated differently by the
OIG depending on their location. For example, an official in the
Washington field office told us that the office would not consider

---

[5]Medicare and Medicaid Patient and Program Protection Act of 1987
(P.L. 100-93).

recommending nationwide exclusion unless the state Medicaid agency had excluded the provider, or a licensing board had revoked a license, for at least 1 year. The Chicago and New York field offices, however, use a 2-year rule of thumb.

OIG NOT NOTIFIED OF CERTAIN WITHDRAWALS FROM STATE MEDICAID PROGRAMS

During our state visits we found that states were not always notifying the OIG of certain providers effectively excluded from the respective state's Medicaid program. One state we visited sometimes permits providers who are being considered for removal from their Medicaid programs to "voluntarily" withdraw rather than face formal sanction. Another state sometimes terminates on short notice providers it suspects of engaging in improper or inappropriate activities. Neither type of withdrawal is reported to the OIG. While this results in safeguards for those states' Medicaid programs and beneficiaries, it affords no protection for Medicare or other states' Medicaid programs.[6]

Illinois sometimes negotiates a settlement agreement with a provider against whom it has initiated termination proceedings. This effectively excludes the provider without the state having to spend the time and resources needed to pursue a formal action. In such an agreement, the provider admits to no wrongdoing but agrees to withdraw from participating in Medicaid. The provider also forfeits the right to appeal if denied reinstatement at a later date. The provider does not, however, face the prospect of losing his or her license to practice because, according to state Medicaid officials, the case is not referred to the state licensing board. In addition, the state does not report such a case to the OIG. This withdrawal process enables Illinois to remove providers from its Medicaid program relatively quickly and keep them out. But, because the state does not report these actions to the state licensing board or the OIG, the providers may continue to provide harmful, unnecessary, or excessive services to beneficiaries in other federal or state programs.

---

[6]Section 1902 of the Social Security Act requires the state Medicaid agency to report to HHS whenever a provider of services is terminated, suspended, or otherwise sanctioned or prohibited from participating in the program. HHS regulations define the term "otherwise sanctioned" as intending to cover all actions that limit the ability of a person to participate in the program regardless of what such an action is called, including situations in which an individual or entity voluntarily withdraws from a program to avoid a formal sanction (42 C.F.R. 1001.601). Furthermore, the provision regarding exclusion for loss of license also defines surrender of license to avoid an adverse action as grounds for exclusion.

Currently, about 23 percent of the physicians not allowed to participate in the Illinois Medicaid program have withdrawn in lieu of an action against them. We found that some of the providers who had withdrawn for what appeared to be serious quality of care problems were still able to bill Medicare in Illinois. For example, Medicare paid a podiatrist over $20,000 for services provided to program beneficiaries since he withdrew from the Illinois Medicaid program in August 1995. The podiatrist withdrew from the program after the state alleged that he had provided grossly inferior care to Medicaid recipients.

An Illinois Medicaid official told us that he did not believe that the settlement agreements preclude the state from formally referring withdrawals to outside organizations. If the state agency started to do so, however, he believed that providers would soon opt to pursue the formal sanction route rather than withdrawing. Consequently, the state might lose a valuable tool for removing undesirable providers from Medicaid and would be forced to spend more time pursuing exclusion. This official speculated that had Illinois not aggressively moved to remove these providers from the Medicaid program through voluntary withdrawals, the providers would still be in the program.

We do not know how prevalent voluntary withdrawals are nationwide. Most of the other states we visited told us they do not allow providers to withdraw from their programs to avoid formal sanction. Although New York sometimes allows providers to withdraw from its program, state Medicaid officials told us these cases are reported to the OIG, the state licensing board, and others. Certain providers New York suspects of abuse, however, are terminated but not reported to the OIG.

We were informed by New York officials that state program regulations permit either the provider or state Medicaid agency to terminate a provider's participation in the program upon 30 days' written notice. According to state officials, this practice has been used primarily against pharmacies that the state suspected were heavily involved in dispensing drugs with a street market. As a result, the state agency has been able to deal quickly with pharmacies that it believed were involved in drug diversion. Like voluntary withdrawals in Illinois, however, these cases are not reported to the OIG.

STATES' USE OF THE OIG'S EXCLUDED PROVIDER LISTS

The OIG widely disseminates information on excluded providers through monthly reports and periodic cumulative listings to various state and federal agencies so that they, too, will remove these providers from their programs. We found, however, that for several reasons states sometimes have difficulty identifying and excluding providers who appear on the lists.

First, the states have difficulty identifying individuals--
such as nurses, pharmacists, or physicians--who are employed by
hospitals, nursing homes, pharmacies, and health maintenance
organizations that bill the program under the entities' billing
number. These providers, once sanctioned, can change employers or
move to other states and potentially continue to provide services
through federal health care programs without detection.

Second, providers sometimes are not identified because states
tend to use the OIG's monthly list for a onetime check against
their active provider files. However, they may not review prior
monthly lists to check a provider who applies for program
participation in a subsequent month. Thus, a provider could later
enroll in the state's Medicaid program after being excluded
nationwide by the OIG and not be detected.

Finally, some states do not always check providers appearing
on the list who have out-of-state addresses. An official in
Missouri, for example, told us that although they check the OIG
monthly list with in-state and border state addresses, they do not
check names from other states. New York officials also told us
that it would be time-consuming to check the list of their Medicaid
providers against the entire OIG list each month; instead, they
only check for New York addresses. In addition, they said the
OIG's cumulative list is cumbersome to use and the information is
not formatted in a way that would permit a large state, such as New
York, to match provider names.

When we performed a computer match of the OIG exclusion list
to Illinois' enrolled provider file, we found 13 out-of-state
providers who had been excluded by the OIG between 1988 and 1995
but who were still enrolled in the Illinois Medicaid program. One
of them had received almost $25,000 in Medicaid payments since
being excluded by the OIG. Although the others had not billed the
program since they were excluded by the OIG, state Medicaid
officials acknowledged that they would have been paid had they
submitted claims.

MAGNITUDE OF PROBLEM
COULD NOT BE DETERMINED

Although we attempted to identify the magnitude and
pervasiveness of problems in the exclusion process, we were unable
to do so--primarily because of a lack of case file documentation at
the OIG field offices.

In our visits to OIG field offices, we found that they were
not always able to fully account for the number of referrals they
received from the states. For example, the Chicago field office
could not locate 5 of 17 referrals sent by a state Medicaid agency
during 1994 and 1995. As a result, it could not confirm that it

had received the referrals or explain why it had not considered exclusion.

Our review of these five cases at the state Medicaid agency determined that three of them involved what appeared to be serious quality of care issues. For example, in April 1995, the Illinois Medicaid agency excluded a dentist from its program for providing care that placed his patients at risk of harm. Among the charges was that the dentist had performed surgical extractions and had given patients general anesthesia without documented need. The state Medicaid agency's case file on this dentist showed that he had been referred to the OIG in June 1995. When we inquired at the Chicago field office in March 1996, however, no record could be found of the case. Subsequent to our inquiry, the office opened a case file on the dentist, but as of August 8, 1996, the case had not been forwarded to headquarters for a final decision. Since this dentist was excluded from Medicaid, he has received almost $12,000 for services provided to Medicare patients.

When discussing weaknesses in the OIG's exclusion process with headquarters officials, they acknowledged that improvements are needed and informed us of a recent initiative to increase the number and quality of exclusion cases being forwarded from the field offices. In May 1996, the OIG began an effort to identify all mandatory exclusion cases referred to them by the states, along with permissive exclusion cases meeting certain criteria. Staff performing this function will receive extra training on the processing of provider exclusions submitted by state agencies.

OIG officials also attributed these problems to resource cuts over the last several years. With the recent enactment of the Health Insurance Portability and Accountability Act of 1996, officials believe they will be able to obtain additional resources to further address these problems.

OBSERVATIONS

Our work to date shows that the opportunity exists for--and indeed we found cases in which--providers deemed to be unfit to participate in one state's Medicaid program can continue to do so in Medicare or in other states. Because of the amount of communication and coordination that is needed at the state and federal levels, the referral and exclusion process is complex. Nevertheless, we believe that more attention must be paid to a system that works to protect beneficiaries from substandard care and helps ensure the integrity of federal health programs.

Although the OIG believes its initiatives and the potential for additional investigative resources will help remedy weaknesses in the long term, we believe that the OIG could take immediate action in several areas that would substantially improve its effectiveness. For example, the OIG could provide more guidance

for OIG field staff and the states to facilitate the prompt
preparation of case files--including required documentation--for
OIG decisions. It could also clarify guidance for the field
offices to ensure more consistency in the cases that are sent
forward to headquarters for a final decision. Furthermore, it
could explore ways to ensure that states quickly identify and act
to remove OIG-excluded providers from Medicaid participation.
Finally, the OIG may want to ask states to begin reporting
information on those who have agreed to withdraw from a state
Medicaid program rather than subject themselves to the formal
sanction process.

- - - - -

Mr. Chairman, this concludes my statement. I would be happy
to respond to any questions that you or Members of the Subcommittee
may have.

For more information on this testimony, please call Kathy Allen,
Assistant Director, at (202) 512-7059. Other major contributors
included Jon Barker, Bob Ferschl, Bob Lippencott, Al Schnupp, and
Ted Wagner.

SECTIONS OF THE SOCIAL SECURITY ACT
UNDER WHICH EXCLUSIONS ARE IMPOSED

Section	Exclusion
1128(a)(1)	Program-related conviction
1128(a)(2)	Conviction for patient abuse or neglect
1128(b)(1)	Conviction related to health care fraud (non-HHS)
1128(b)(2)	Conviction related to obstruction of an investigation
1128(b)(3)	Conviction related to controlled substances
1128(b)(4)	License revocation or suspension
1128(b)(5)	Suspension or exclusion under a federal or state health care program
1128(b)(6)	Excessive claims or furnishing of unnecessary or substandard items and services
1128(b)(7)	Fraud, kickbacks, and other related activities
1128(b)(8)	Entities owned or controlled by a sanctioned individual
1128(b)(9)	Failure to disclose required information
1128(b)(10)	Failure to supply requested information on subcontractors and suppliers
1128(b)(11)	Failure to provide payment information
1128(b)(12)	Failure to grant immediate access
1128(b)(13)	Failure to take corrective action
1128(b)(14)	Default on health education loan or scholarship obligations
1128Aa	Imposition of a civil money penalty or assessment
1156(b)	Peer review organization recommendation

(101503)

Mr. SHAYS. Thank you very much. Mr. Souder.

Mr. SOUDER. One of the questions that I had was, in this lag time from the time somebody is being investigated to the time that they're excluded, is there not a suspension; in other words, where they can't continue to provide services?

Ms. ARONOVITZ. There is very strong concern about due process. And the cases that we're talking about are not even ones where the provider is under investigation.

We're talking about time delays even after the person has already been convicted in a State court. It could be for program-related fraud or patient abuse or neglect.

It's even after these cases that the person has been convicted the process works so that the OIG field office is notified, and that's where a lot of the delays are.

Mr. SOUDER. A lot of the delays? You had a couple of really egregious cases.

Ms. ARONOVITZ. Let me clarify that. We don't really know the extent of the problem. One of the reasons is that when we went to the OIG field offices, what we wanted to do was obtain a universe of all referrals that were made to the OIG field office. We could then look and see how many cases were handled quickly and do a time line to see how many cases were, in fact, delayed for unreasonable lengths of time.

In the case of the OIG field offices, when a case was referred to an OIG field office at the places we went to and know action was going to be taken—in other words, at the field office there was a determination that the case would not go forward—it was destroyed.

There was no record or log or no historical data kept that that case was ever even received in the field office. So we could never get a universe of cases that the OIG field office had received.

Mr. SOUDER. I'm doubling back, because that seems like something fairly obvious that needs to be addressed.

In the question of due process, when it may even be that the State and Federal are both investigating somebody, is there either a lot of cases like that that are pending investigations, or would there be a way to have a preliminary hearing where you would say this looks like this one may go forward, as opposed to being a harassing charge or just an individual filed a complaint, where there is enough reason to believe?

Because I would guess that that's where there may even be more cases than in the other.

Ms. ARONOVITZ. That's a very tricky issue, I would think, because people are under investigation all the time from very many different sources—Medicaid Fraud Control Units.

The licensing board sometimes is investigating someone for licensing action, and also the Medicaid agencies themselves and also the OIG, the U.S. attorney's office.

When there is suspicion of inadequate care or substandard care or program integrity violations, there is a lot of concern about identifying a provider as a bad provider when, in fact, it will turn out that the court doesn't, in fact, declare him as such.

So I think there would be a lot of concern on the part of State and Federal officials about taking premature action in those cases.

Mr. SOUDER. I can understand why there would be that concern. At the same time, when you look at the balance, that's a lot how the regular legal system works.

There is charges filed. Then, if you go forward with an indictment, often somebody is let go from their job or temporarily on leave or you don't do business with somebody. And then, the final termination comes at conviction.

And it seems like there is a window here, if this goes on, like you say, for an extended period of time, where literally the taxpayers could be getting drained in all 50 States simultaneously.

Ms. ARONOVITZ. You're correct. I think the IG and probably some of the State people could probably elaborate on your question even more.

I would imagine also that if there was some indication of egregious action, there would be some process to eliminate that person from practicing or taking some licensing action immediately. I'm not that familiar with it, and I'm sure someone else could address that.

But we're talking even about cases where someone gets convicted. We're finding that those people continue to practice in Medicare or other Federal programs, and that's really scary to us.

Mr. SOUDER. And that's, kind of, step one, where you think you'd be able to continue to catch that.

Ms. ARONOVITZ. Exactly.

Mr. SOUDER. How difficult is the problem? I mean, maybe because not that many people are being caught that it isn't even that big a pressure, but as we would get better systems and start to crack down, how easy and what methods could be taken to keep people from transferring their addresses, the principal in one group becoming a secondary person in another but providing the expertise on how to cheat the Government? How would you begin to sort through that process?

Ms. ARONOVITZ. That's a very, very large and complex question. A lot of people have talked about using a universal or unique provider identification number. Individuals would hold onto that number for their whole careers and couldn't continue to hide under entity billing numbers and all.

There are a lot of different initiatives. There used to be the PIN in Medicare, and then they went to the UPIN with COBRA in 1985, and that was an effort to try to establish a unique physician identification number for all Medicare physicians.

Now, with the Medicare Transaction System, the national provider identifier, which is an NPI—it's another acronym—but it's another attempt to try to assure that all Medicare providers use the same number for their career and bill all Medicare carriers for those same services under that same number, and that also would be their billing number.

So there are a lot of attempts at trying to get to this problem. We're not there yet or anywhere close. The Kennedy-Kassebaum bill also provides for different types of identifiers that I could discuss later, if you'd like, or elaborate, if you'd like.

Mr. SOUDER. Thank you.

Mr. SHAYS. Thank you. Mr. Towns.

Mr. TOWNS. Thank you very much, Mr. Chairman. Looking at the chart there, regarding those exclusion leads, let me ask the question what recommendations would you make to achieve consistency, considering the various areas of exclusion leads? Could you make some specific recommendations?

Ms. ARONOVITZ. Well, the eight OIG field offices receive referrals, as this chart shows, from many, many different sources, one of which is the Medicaid office.

It is our understanding that a lot of the leads that the OIG receives are not anything that they really can act on.

In fact, some of the leads come from organizations at the State level, where the OIG doesn't even have any jurisdiction.

Mr. TOWNS. That's correct.

Ms. ARONOVITZ. And what we would hope is that the OIG field office staff would be sufficiently trained, and they would understand exactly what the jurisdiction was of the OIG. And they would be able to screen these referrals so that they would know which ones to pursue and spend time with.

There are a lot of things that could be screened out at the OIG field office because States very often don't prescreen referrals.

They'll just send everything. Like all licensing action, for instance, from the licensing board, they'll send it to the OIG, much of which the OIG wouldn't really be in a position to deal with.

For instance, if a license was suspended for 3 months, by the time the OIG would evaluate the facts in the case and try to make a decision and get it to headquarters, the suspension would be over.

That person would be reinstated, and then it would be a matter of them trying to get off an OIG exclusion list, so there are certain guidelines that the OIG has.

So I think the first line of defense would be for the OIG field offices to do a really good job in screening the referrals they get to assure that the ones that they concentrate on are ones that are either mandatory exclusions because they're convictions of health care fraud, related fraud or patient abuse, or ones that are permissive that have such a high level of evidence that it would be incumbent upon the OIG to consider it.

Mr. TOWNS. Right. Are you familiar with Project WEED?

Ms. ARONOVITZ. Yes. Yes, I am.

Mr. TOWNS. Will that get us there?

Ms. ARONOVITZ. I think Project WEED is a great attempt to start backing up a little bit and then going forward in terms of understanding what is out there and what the OIG has missed in the past.

I think Ms. Brown will explain that last November we've seen some documents that—in the spring talk about going back and identifying cases in the OIG field offices that were mandatory exclusion referrals that were never sent to headquarters.

And I think they're doing an excellent job now of trying to go back and identify those cases and take action on them. But a lot of this depends on how consistent and comprehensive this effort is in the future to decide whether it would be effective.

I think the most important thing is that the OIG have the people in the field offices that understand how the system works; they're committed to it and it's a high enough priority that the resources are there for them to be able to pursue this.

Mr. TOWNS. Right. You wanted to add something, Ms. Allen? Oh, I thought you wanted to jump in here.

When I look at this chart, I can see a lot of problems, because when you talk about authority, you do have licensing boards.

I mean, everybody is involved here, and I just, sort of, wonder if you had any kind of specific ideas or recommendations, because you have State legislators that would be involved in many States.

So I was just trying to figure out if you had any kind of specific suggestions or recommendations that we could come up with that we could put into legislation in terms of bringing about some consistency.

As the chairman indicated earlier, this is a committee. We're not having these hearings just to have hearings. We're serious about trying to do something about this problem. And when I look at that chart, I can see there are a lot of problems.

Ms. ARONOVITZ. One of the options that the OIG might have is to work with the States to be much more specific with the States about what they refer up.

Now, that doesn't mean the States are going to listen. It's very time-consuming for a State licensing board to separate its list based on all the actions it took and those that they think that the OIG would need to act on.

The one area that I think would be pretty clear and straightforward might be those that involve a conviction for a mandatory exclusion case, that those maybe should be sent up separately or sent up for sure and the other ones.

The OIG I think is going to have to work with the States. It's going to take a lot of cajoling, I think, in negotiating in terms of trying to get States to do a little bit of a better job in screening the referrals that come to the OIG.

It's a tough question, and it is a lot of work for the OIG field offices to ferret through that.

Mr. TOWNS. But you do agree that the lack of uniformity among States is very significant?

Ms. ARONOVITZ. Yes, I do, but it extends further than that. I think it extends to the lack of uniformity even among the field offices in terms of what they look at as being serious enough to consider.

So there is a real opportunity for guidance on both the State and the Federal OIG field office level.

Mr. TOWNS. Thank you very much. Thank you, Mr. Chairman.

Mr. SHAYS. I thank the gentleman. We have some seats in the front row that are really not reserved for anyone. If any of you would like to come up to the——

Mr. SCHIFF. Mr. Chairman, that group is waiting for me.

Mr. SHAYS. Oh, OK.

Mr. SCHIFF. Thank you for that courtesy.

Mr. SHAYS. OK.

Mr. SCHIFF. I'm waiting to see if you're going to call on me or call on yourself next.

Mr. SHAYS. I'm going to call on you, sir. You don't come in late and call on yourself first.

Mr. SCHIFF. Mr. Chairman, you're the chairman. You can do whatever you want.

Mr. SHAYS. When I believe that, then I'm dead.

Mr. SCHIFF. Ms. Aronovitz, what are the three most important things that could be done at any level of government to solve the problem of people remaining eligible for being paid Medicare services or Medicaid services, whatever, health care services, when, in fact, they really ought to be removed from all programs?

What would you list the top three things that could be done, even if we can't do them all here in Congress?

Ms. ARONOVITZ. I think it's very important to make sure that State organizations, State agencies, are identifying and referring to the OIG those people that have committed the most egregious either crimes or situations.

Mr. SCHIFF. Reporting is No. 1?

Ms. ARONOVITZ. The first one is to identify and try, if possible, and it's not that easy, to try to get the States to weed through all the referrals they make and identify those that are the most compelling. And those would be the ones that have a mandatory exclusion responsibility.

There are now four statutes that require automatic exclusion from all Federal programs, health care programs, if the person is convicted of those four statutes. It's very straightforward. It's not that difficult.

Mr. SCHIFF. And we need to identify and report that to the OIG.

Ms. ARONOVITZ. To the OIG.

Mr. SCHIFF. OK.

Ms. ARONOVITZ. Right. That's No. 1.

Mr. SCHIFF. No. 1.

Ms. ARONOVITZ. The second is for the OIG to figure out how to streamline its system so that people at the regional levels are knowledgeable and have the resources to quickly and accurately report this information to headquarters, knowing that every day they wait a provider—we have one example where a provider drilled through a child's cheek in the process of giving him some dental care. I mean, this is a disaster.

This person was immediately excluded from a State Medicaid program, and it took 5 years for the licensing board to get around to taking the person on probation and then finally revoking the license and then finally getting the person referred to the OIG so that the OIG could take action.

So it's to get these cases. Every day that you wait, you know that there is a chance that beneficiaries are very much at risk, and also, the program's integrity.

So it's to realize that this is a very high priority, figure out how to streamline the system so that the cases get reviewed immediately and then are sent to the headquarters for final decision.

Mr. SCHIFF. That's No. 2?

Ms. ARONOVITZ. That's No. 2, I would say. And then, the third one would be to figure out how to get the information on the OIG exclusion list out to as many people as easily and carefully as possible.

And that involves making sure that list is comprehensive, that it's accurate and that it gives as much information as possible so that as many people who access that list could use it in a way that doesn't end up being very cumbersome.

For instance, when you have a list of 8,800 providers and it's on the Internet, that's a wonderful thing. However, it's still very cumbersome to manually check the names on the list. You have to do computer matches without any kind of complete identification numbers.

We have a situation where we tried to do some matching and found we got a ton of hits, but it turns out that it was based on names. We didn't have a provider number to compare to. So we could not definitively identify a particular person.

Mr. SCHIFF. There might be more than one Dr. John Smith.

Ms. ARONOVITZ. Right. Did you want to elaborate on that, Bob? You did some of the matches.

Mr. FERSCHL. When we tried to do matches, particularly between States or between the IG's list and State enrollment files, we did run into that problem because we had missing identifiers or because States use different identifying systems than the IG did.

And when we tried to do this matching, we did it by name, and like you said, there are a lot of John Smiths, and you get a lot of erroneous matches. They're very time consuming to resolve.

Ms. ARONOVITZ. And it would really be a terrible disservice to a provider who is doing a good job to subject him to this kind of process, if it wasn't the right provider.

Mr. SCHIFF. I thank you very much. I yield back, Mr. Chairman.

Mr. SHAYS. Could I just have you reiterate your three?

Ms. ARONOVITZ. Sure. I think the first one has to do with States identifying, weeding through their referrals and making sure that they refer the most severe cases to the IG; the OIG system having the resources and the process in place to be able to quickly act on them.

It's not that difficult, if you have the resources and you have the knowledge on how to do this. And the third one is to figure out how to make the notification process more simple for States.

Mr. SHAYS. Thank you. Mr. Green.

Mr. GREEN. Thank you, Mr. Chairman. First of all, I'd like to compliment the chairman and the ranking member because, in the Portability Act that was just signed, there were some reforms in there.

And are you familiar enough with what was put in by the chairman to comment on them today and see where it's at in the program?

Ms. ARONOVITZ. I think so.

Mr. GREEN. And another thing, for a provider to be excluded from Medicaid reimbursement or payments, they don't also have to lose their license to practice?

Ms. ARONOVITZ. That's correct.

Mr. GREEN. OK.

Ms. ARONOVITZ. In many cases, a State will exclude them from Medicaid even though they don't lose their license. But once they are excluded from Medicaid, the State would then refer that provider to the State licensing board, and the State licensing board could decide whether it wanted to take separate action.

You also have a situation of people who voluntarily withdraw from the Medicaid Program when they know they're going to have to face formal sanctions.

In those cases, usually, or at least in the State we were in where this happens, the agreement to withdraw specifies that they won't tell the licensing board. So it, kind of, gives the State some leverage to get them out of Medicaid quickly.

Mr. GREEN. I just know typically, in the dental example you made, because of due process requirements—and we don't want to change that—it's almost impossible to take a professional license, except for lawyers.

I see it every month that lawyers lose their license, but I also know the process to take a professional license is, you're right, 5 years may be a short time in some cases.

But can you comment on the changes of the provisions that were in the Portability Act that may address some of the concerns of the study that you did?

Ms. ARONOVITZ. Sure. Sure. There is, actually, two major areas where I think the act could help this process.

One of them has to do with the establishment of the adverse action data bank. Theoretically, setting up the adverse action data bank really gets to some of the problems that we talk about.

However, there are a lot of concerns in terms of implementation that we would still have in terms of how this data bank gets implemented.

No. 1, the data bank itself requires that there be a taxpayer identification number and a name attached to every provider that gets input into the system.

However, as I said before, some States use a—it's called a TIN, taxpayer identification number. In different States, you could use different TIN's. You could use an employee identification number. Some States let you use a Social Security number.

The first concern we had would be that there might be an insufficient amount of information put into the data base that identifies the person. So that States would have trouble doing their matches or identifying the correct person.

You'd also have the problem with unenrolled providers. As I mentioned earlier, there are nurses who work in nursing homes, physicians who work in hospitals and HMO's, and pharmacists who work in pharmacies who do not bill under their own number.

So that the entity billing could still hire an excluded provider, and they might not get detected even though their name was in this adverse action data bank.

There are some other implementation issues. We'd want to make sure that the data bank had accurate and complete information, which is not an easy task, when you're asking all these different parties to put in information.

I mean, we looked a little bit at some of the lessons that are being learned in the National Practitioners Data Bank.

And one of the things we're hearing is that a lot, a lot of people want to retrieve information from that data bank that has to do with licensing actions and sanctions and hospital sanctions.

A lot of people want to retrieve from it, but not that many people input into it. So it's a very, very tricky situation to keep this data bank accurate and up to date, especially for people who get reinstated, because you don't want it to be easy to access their names if, in fact, they're no longer, out of the program.

One other thing that we're concerned about besides protections, in terms of who could access this, and I'm sure that would be worked out, but there is one gap or one area in the law, in the adverse action data bank, and that is that it says that all final adverse actions must be submitted to the data bank.

But what it says also is that a settlement that involved no findings of liability does not have to be included. In other words, a settlement that has no findings of a liability is not considered to be a final adverse action and would not have to be in the data bank.

So the case I described earlier where you have a voluntary withdrawal—somebody gets nervous, they think they're going to end up being convicted of something, they voluntarily withdraw from Medicaid—their names would not be in this data bank.

The one thing I do want to say about the TIN, and this is the other part of the Kennedy-Kassebaum Act, is that it addresses another type of number, and it's called a UHI, a unique health identifier, and that's under the administrative simplification section of the act.

And it says that all patients, providers and all different other types of billing entities would have this number.

We think that number really gets much closer to what you would probably need to be able to have the adverse action data bank work. So you'd have to reconcile the requirement for a TIN that's currently in the data bank section and instead maybe replace it with the UHI.

The one big problem with the UHI is that that is going to take quite a while for it to be implemented. So it's several years down the road we think before every provider has that number and is using it in billing all the different programs.

Theoretically, it's taking us much closer, but there are still a lot of challenges ahead.

Mr. GREEN. Thank you, Mr. Chairman.

Mr. SHAYS. I thank the gentleman. I'd like to just be clear on a few general issues. One is I'm having a hard time sorting out—I mean, the more I think about it the harder I am trying to sort it out.

And that is that we're not just dealing with 50 plus State agencies and territories, obviously, but we're dealing with the contractors, say, for Medicaid and Medicare as well. When you have a number, who gives you the number?

Ms. ARONOVITZ. It's a very complex story. And, in fact, there are a lot of different numbers. There are, actually, about six or seven different efforts to try to make numbers more uniform. Three deal with Medicare, and some of them I talked about.

Maybe, if I could, just go through some of these, you could see how difficult it is to try to get to a "uniform" or a unique identifier.

In Medicare, there would be a PIN, a Provider Identification Number, for each specific carrier, and then there was a separate billing number.

Mr. SHAYS. By carrier, you mean the person paying the bill?

Ms. ARONOVITZ. Right. In Medicare, each carrier issued a separate PIN, and it was easy to get multiple billing numbers. It was easy to get these numbers. After COBRA 85——

Mr. SHAYS. Let me just tell you I don't need a history.

Ms. ARONOVITZ. OK.

Mr. SHAYS. Tell me right now what the process is.

Ms. ARONOVITZ. The process would be that every 1 of the 50 States in Medicaid could still use their own system for giving a provider a Medicaid number.

Mr. SHAYS. So the States give the number?

Ms. ARONOVITZ. In Medicaid, the States would give the numbers.

Mr. SHAYS. OK.

Ms. ARONOVITZ. Now, in Medicare, the UPIN is the effort that's most underway, except that with the Medicare Transaction System, we're headed toward the National Provider Identifier, which will probably take the place of the UPIN, and it will incorporate a lot more types of providers. I know this is very complicated.

Mr. SHAYS. I'm a reasonable man.

Ms. ARONOVITZ. Well, it's very interesting, because when people talk about wanting a uniform provider number, it sounds so simple, but there are quite a lot of——

Mr. SHAYS. First off, just tell me who gives the numbers. I'll start from that.

Ms. ARONOVITZ. OK.

Mr. SHAYS. The States give the Medicaid numbers?

Ms. ARONOVITZ. Right. And in Medicare, the——

Mr. SHAYS. The contractors?

Ms. ARONOVITZ. The contractors, right.

Mr. SHAYS. OK. And how many contractors are we talking about? I don't mind if you want to turn to either side here, because I really want to nail this down a bit.

Ms. ALLEN. I believe there are 70 carriers and intermediaries now. But again, under MTS, there is an attempt to consolidate that and to establish a single UPIN or the——

Ms. ARONOVITZ. NPI.

Ms. ALLEN [continuing]. NPI that one can use for all of their billing.

Ms. ARONOVITZ. Right, for part A and part B, for all the carriers, for the whole Medicare Program.

Mr. SHAYS. In our legislation, we're directing the Secretary to work toward a unified number.

Ms. ARONOVITZ. Right.

Mr. SHAYS. But I'm really trying to get a handle on whose toes we step on in terms of that process. For instance, I'd love to know how long it took us to do, but we got this out of the computer. This is the exclusionary list, and frankly, it's quite impressive.

I mean, we, basically, put together a book, but having done that, I'm not quite sure how helpful it is. I'm trying to get a handle on that, but it just seems to me that you should need a number to do business in Medicare and Medicaid and CHAMPUS.

And it would strike me that it should be, ideally, one number.

Ms. ARONOVITZ. Right.

Mr. SHAYS. And then the question is who gives the number. We have to, Republicans and Democrats, have to realize that when we do certain things, we can't have it both ways.

We do want local governments and State governments. We, the majority party, want local and State governments to run programs as best as possible.

But we now established a Federal law establishing health care fraud as a Federal offense, an all-payer, public and private. That's what we've done.

So we're having the Federal Government step in, and obviously, it's our money. So we're trying to see how this marries, but it seems to me that you should get one number. And if you don't have a number, you don't do business.

Ms. ARONOVITZ. In the act, in this new act, the UHI, the Unique Health Identifier, I think really gets to your concern.

It's going to, hopefully, cover all different types of providers and people who participate in all different types of programs. Right now, it's in its early stages. The bill just passed.

There is a lot of work that needs to be done. We're way off, but I think that will get to, ultimately, where I think you're headed.

Mr. SHAYS. One of the things that didn't get in the legislation was that we wanted to hold liable the contractors and those that authorize the payment for someone who was on the list. I mean, if they didn't check the list, then they paid it out. That's one problem.

One problem is where you're on the list and you're still getting paid. That's an absurdity.

Ms. ARONOVITZ. Right.

Mr. SHAYS. But then there are other people who should be on the list, and the process takes too long. And then there are people who are on that list but have another number, and they're just actively playing another program. So I guess we got a ways to go.

Ms. ARONOVITZ. Right. I think HCFA is here. They're eminently qualified to talk about the Medicare numbers and all that, but I think, really, the UHI I think is getting closer than we've been before, at least theoretically.

Mr. SHAYS. But we're, potentially, talking about lots of doctors.

Ms. ARONOVITZ. Absolutely.

Mr. SHAYS. And hospitals and nurses and so on.

Ms. ARONOVITZ. Right.

Mr. SHAYS. Some of whom have done outrageous things.

Ms. ARONOVITZ. Right.

Mr. SHAYS. And we have some who have defrauded the system for millions and millions of dollars. So there is a gigantic incentive to not only get closer but to get closer a lot sooner than we have.

Ms. ARONOVITZ. Absolutely.

Mr. SHAYS. And this is an effort that we want to work with you and both sides of the aisle, because it's just a win for all of us, if we can.

I'm going to defer my other questions for other witnesses, but let me just ask both of your colleagues what would you add to that list of three that we have so far?

Mr. FERSCHL. I think that that would pretty well cover it. I think those are the three——

Mr. SHAYS. Were you tempted to suggest another one, I mean, if you had a fourth or fifth? I won't say that you're replacing her one, two, or three.

Mr. FERSCHL. Offhand, nothing comes to mind.

Mr. SHAYS. Ms. Allen.

Ms. ALLEN. Likewise, none off the top of my head, sir.

Mr. SHAYS. OK. Do any of the Members have followup questions before we get to the next panel?

[No response.]

Mr. SHAYS. We thank you very much. Our next panel is June Gibbs Brown, the inspector general of the Department of Health and Human Services, and then Judy Berek, the senior advisor, program integrity for Health Care Financing Administration, HCFA.

We'll go first with June Gibbs Brown. And I'd ask you both to remain standing. If you'd please raise your right hands. We swear in all our witnesses, including Members of Congress.

[Witnesses sworn.]

Mr. SHAYS. For the record, both witnesses have responded in the affirmative. I think, Ms. Brown, we'll begin with you.

We have the 5-minute rule, but it's important that you make your testimony as you want to, and so we'll let you go over.

STATEMENTS OF JUNE GIBBS BROWN, INSPECTOR GENERAL, DEPARTMENT OF HEALTH AND HUMAN SERVICES; AND JUDY BEREK, SENIOR ADVISOR, PROGRAM INTEGRITY, HEALTH CARE FINANCING ADMINISTRATION

Ms. BROWN. Thank you, Mr. Chairman, and members of the subcommittee. I'm June Gibbs Brown, inspector general of the U.S. Department of Health and Human Services.

My written testimony addresses your specific questions about the length of time it takes to exclude those providers from Medicare that States have already excluded from Medicaid, the form and usefulness of information provided to the States on exclusion cases, and the effectiveness of the permissive exclusions.

Over the years, the OIG has made substantial progress with regard to the exclusion process, but we recognize that more is needed.

We expect to exclude about 1,500 providers by the end of this fiscal year. As of July 31, we had implemented 1,237 exclusions of which 463 were mandatory and 774 were permissive.

Despite a 50-percent reduction in our investigative staff since 1992, the OIG implemented an average of 1,200 new exclusions annually, and fewer than 1 percent of these OIG-imposed exclusions have ever been overturned on appeal.

When I became inspector general at the end of 1993, I determined to improve the exclusion process. One of the first things I did was to rescind an earlier directive to suspend the screening and processing of certain categories of exclusion leads.

That directive had been issued because of the budget constraints that limited the OIG's ability to act in the area.

I also set goals to improve the methods by which we report exclusion actions to governmental and private entities and to the public.

The reporting mechanisms are important because once the OIG excludes a provider, the key to enforcing the exclusion is good communication.

My written testimony describes the many types of hard copy and electronic notices and listings the OIG routinely provides within the health care payer network.

In addition, lists of excluded individuals and entities are available to governmental agencies and the general public on the Internet. Information on how to access the World Wide Web site is attached to my written testimony.

I also asked my staff to step up their educational outreach to reporting entities on the type of documentation we need in order to take action on a case at a national level.

For example, the OIG staff recently participated in an annual conference of the National Association of Surveillance Officials and conducted extensive sanction training for Medicare contractors in the New York and Boston regions.

My staff met with GAO representatives on several occasions in recent weeks to discuss their observations and recommendations, and we are in general agreement with them.

We are giving priority attention to GAO's concern about tracking incoming exclusion leads, and we now maintain a data base of incoming referrals.

The OIG's past procedures evolved out of a complex operational environment in which exclusion leads not only from the State Medicaid agencies but from many other sources in each of the 50 States flow into eight OIG field offices.

I have with me a chart that illustrates the work flow. The leads referred to the OIG field offices are screened against Federal exclusion criteria, documented, and transmitted to OIG headquarters for appropriate action.

Sometimes, we do not receive the necessary documents from State agencies. There are delays in formal court proceedings, or the OIG cannot act on leads because the State authorities have not taken the final action.

Mr. SHAYS. This is your chart?

Ms. BROWN. Yes.

Mr. SHAYS. Are we to make an assumption that each block is a contact with your office? I mean, frankly, this isn't as clear to me as it may be to some other Members.

Ms. BROWN. All right. In most States——

Mr. SHAYS. I see these blocks just floating, and do they all directly report to——

Ms. BROWN. We get input from any and all of these.

Mr. SHAYS. OK.

Ms. BROWN. Some States don't have all of them. Many States do; also the territories. But all of these entities, and there may be some we've missed, can forward these leads.

Mr. SHAYS. OK.

Ms. BROWN. Sometimes what they give us is just a piece of paper saying somebody was convicted. We can't act on that. We have to have the actual documentation from the courts.

We need to follow certain criteria; and some of these entities are very unresponsive when we try to get back to them. Where we've just had a piece of paper and we can't get additional information, sometimes the lead is discarded.

GAO pointed out to me that they couldn't track these, and I immediately put in a system where we have a data base.

Now all leads, when they come in, no matter how inadequately supported, are immediately put on that data base so we have a tracking system to certify that the proper things are being done.

Mr. SHAYS. Now, the bottom line of this chart is just these are examples of some of the groups that you may have contact with; i.e., leads that you then have to followup on?

Ms. BROWN. That's right.

Mr. SHAYS. OK.

Ms. BROWN. And that's true in all of the States and the territories. So it isn't a matter of just going out to one entity in each State and giving training. This is a very expansive process that we have to go through.

In May of this year, we got our 1996 budget. At that point we began implementing a strategy we developed to shore up our effectiveness on exclusions.

The initiative, called Project WEED, will increase the number and quality of exclusion cases being developed by our field offices.

The project ensures through staff training and improved guidelines that the documents necessary to process these cases are gathered and developed as quickly as possible.

Eight senior program analysts in our investigative field offices are assigned to the project. They underwent intensive sanction training in July and, during July and August, identified over 900 potential exclusions that had not been forwarded to our office.

Research on these leads is ongoing. Eleven additional personnel are scheduled to receive this training the week of September 9.

These steps are in harmony with the GAO recommendations and help resolve shortcomings in the system that we had also identified.

The recent passage and signing of the Health Insurance Portability and Accountability Act of 1996 provides more resources and stronger authorities for the OIG. I believe we are now in a position to make greater progress in excluding bad providers.

We appreciate your continued interest in administrative sanctions and welcome your support in helping us make improvements.

This completes my oral testimony, and I'm happy to answer your questions.

[The prepared statement of Ms. Brown follows:]

Good Morning, Mr. Chairman and members of the Subcommittee. I am June Gibbs Brown, Inspector General of the U.S. Department of Health and Human Services. I am pleased to be here because, for the first time in several years, the OIG is in a position to deal effectively with Medicaid exclusion leads. My testimony will address your questions -- specifically, the length of time it takes to exclude providers from Medicare that States have already excluded from Medicaid; the form and usefulness of information provided to States on exclusion cases; and the effectiveness of permissive exclusions.

I would like to state at the outset that many of the problems cited by GAO are valid despite the progress we have made in this area. The OIG expects to exclude about 1,500 providers by the end of this fiscal year. As of July 31, we had implemented 1,237 exclusions, of which 463 were mandatory and 774 were permissive. We are proud of the fact that fewer than one percent of OIG-imposed exclusions have ever been overturned on appeal.

My staff and I met with GAO representatives on several occasions in recent weeks to discuss their observations and recommendations, and we are in general agreement with them. In May of this year when we got our Fiscal Year 1996 budget, we began implementing a program to shore up our effectiveness on exclusions. We call it Project WEED. In addition, the OIG field offices now maintain a data base on all incoming exclusion leads. We developed Project Weed last November as a strategy to deal with exclusion leads. We began implementation shortly after our funding stabilized. I will explain more about this project later in my testimony.

Support from the Congress

Since your June 1995 hearing on administrative sanctions, your staff and ours have met on several occasions to develop proposals to enhance our ability to get dishonest providers out of the programs. These proposals were reflected in the bills you sponsored along with Congressman Schiff. We particularly urge you to continue to pursue the provision requiring Medicare contractors and State Medicaid agencies to be fiscally liable for payments they make to excluded providers. I would also like to mention that we met with Congressman Towns' staff and appreciate his support on these issues as well.

The recent passage and signing of the Health Insurance Portability and Accountability Act of 1996 (Public Law 104-191) provides more resources and stronger authorities for the OIG. Therefore, we are now in a position to make greater progress in excluding bad providers and in precluding inappropriate payment to them.

The Operational Environment

I would like to describe the operational environment in which exclusion leads are processed and some of the challenges we face. We are giving priority attention to GAO's concern about tracking incoming exclusion leads. The current lack of uniformity evolved out of a complex operational environment in which exclusion leads, not only from the State Medicaid agencies, but from many other sources in each of the 50 States, flow into 8 OIG field offices. The staff time available to develop these leads has been minimal at best; and, at one point in the past, work on certain permissive exclusion leads had to be suspended.

Budget constraints in 1992, prior to my appointment, caused the OIG to reevaluate priorities. Limited funding caused the office to realign field office configurations, removing the OIG presence from some States. At that time, the OIG reviewed the exclusion authorities and decided that OIG resources could be put to better use by not acting on cases where State licensing boards or other Federal/State health care programs had already revoked or suspended licenses or participation privileges and the practitioner continued to live in the State that took the action. The OIG believed the State action protected patients since unlicensed physicians could not treat Medicare or Medicaid patients.

When I became Inspector General in November 1993, I rescinded that directive and ordered that all categories of exclusion leads be screened and processed. We also began expanding the methods by which we report exclusion actions to governmental and private entities and the public. For example, exclusion listings are now available on the Internet. I also asked my staff to increase educational outreach to reporting entities on the type of documentation we need in order to take action on a case at the national level.

Some recent outreach examples include participation in the Twelfth Annual Conference of the National Association of Surveillance Officials and presentations before the New Mexico Medicaid Fraud Control Unit training conference, a joint endeavor across the Medicaid program agencies within that State, as well as extensive sanction training conducted in the New York and Boston regional offices for all Medicare contractors within their jurisdiction.

At present, for each of the 50 States and U.S. Territories, there are individual State agencies overseeing the Medicaid programs, separate Medicaid Fraud Control Units, multiple Medicare contractors processing claims for services provided to Part A and Part B beneficiaries and railroad retirees, Medicare Fraud Control Units, multiple licensing boards, titles V and XX State agencies, as well as Federal and State health care agencies too numerous to categorize. All of these agencies funnel conviction, disciplinary and "lead" information into our field offices. Attached is a chart showing the flow of these multi-source leads through our field offices for development and then into headquarters for appropriate action.

Although there are newer technologies, such as accessible databases, that enable the Federal and State health care agencies and the public and private sectors to communicate in a faster and more meaningful fashion, the problem still remains that many agencies and entities are reporting to our office in traditional and less efficient ways.

I want to emphasize that the OIG has always pursued quality of care cases. Where the patient population was subject to known jeopardy, OIG policy has been to take whatever action is within its scope of authority to bar providers from national programs.

The scope of authority for licensing board actions and other State and Federal program actions (section 1128(b)(4) and (b)(5)) is a key element here. The OIG sometimes cannot act upon referrals because disciplinary actions taken by licensing authorities or other Federal or State agencies may not meet Federal statutory requirements. That is why the OIG treats such reports from other sources as "leads" for potential action. Once it is established that these leads have merit and the potential exists for exclusions to be substantiated, then our field offices are able to act upon the information.

The OIG does not have the authority to act on a national level on a "moral turpitude" finding by the State, on a practitioner's failure to renew his or her license, or on items that are not related to the delivery of a health care item or service, like spousal abuse, vehicular manslaughter, drunken-driving, or failure to make child support payments. Thus, not every referral made to our offices is actionable by the OIG.

This office can act upon violations involving professional performance, professional competence, or financial integrity. However, even when the State's actions do meet our criteria by being related to professional performance, professional competence, or financial integrity, there may be other reasons why we cannot take an exclusion action. For instance, we may only exclude an individual or entity that has been suspended or excluded from participation, or "otherwise sanctioned" in a final action in which the State took a disciplinary action. Interim actions such as probation, fines, or continuing education do not equate to final actions if the subject can continue to practice medicine while meeting the State's restrictions.

The OIG retains the discretionary ability to act upon these cases under the authorities contained in sections 1128(b)(6) and 1156 of the Social Security Act. However, both of these procedures are extremely prolonged and labor intensive. The OIG has devoted the necessary resources to such cases, particularly if they affect quality of care; and they are very time consuming and expensive. Let me give you one example.

- In February 1992, the OIG excluded a California oncologist for 10 years under section 1128(b)(6)(B) because the OIG determined that he had rendered over 3,900 excessive, substandard, unnecessary, and potentially risky services to seven Medicare beneficiaries over a six-year period of time. Subsequent to that exclusion, the peer review organization (PRO) submitted two separate recommendations that this same doctor be excluded under section 1156 because he had failed to comply substantially with his obligations in the care of six Medicare beneficiaries with 10 hospital admissions. This care was found to have included, among other violations, inappropriate blood transfusion, inappropriate treatment for sepsis, and failure to detect the development of a decubitus ulcer while the patient was under medical care during a prolonged hospitalization. In August 1992, the OIG acted on the PRO's recommendation and excluded the doctor for another 10 years to run concurrently with the first exclusion. After a lengthy and extremely costly hearing, the administrative law judge upheld the OIG's exclusion actions and determined that the exclusion should be permanent.

Although the State licensing authority and various payer agencies had been investigating this physician for many years without successful result, the OIG took the lead in implementing disciplinary action. However, once the exclusion was in place, the licensing board did revoke the doctor's license. Then it stayed the revocation and put the license on probation. The stay has since been lifted but if the OIG had not devoted its investigative power, resources, and financial backing to excluding this physician, the Medicare/Medicaid patient population would have continued to be at grave risk during the four years that the licensing board took to get to an exclusionable point in its process.

Communication--The Key to Success

When an exclusion is imposed, the OIG makes every effort to publicize it. We send individual notification letters with the subject's personal identifier information (i.e., social security number, date of birth, unique physician identification number (UPIN), program provider number, license number, etc.) to all of the State agencies, Medicare contractors, licensing board, and any known employer in the State where the subject practices medicine. We also send copies of the exclusion notice to the subject's attorney (if known), the Public Health Service, Department of Justice, U.S. Attorney, and any peer review organization that may be deemed appropriate.

Monthly, we notify payer agencies of the exclusions being implemented; specific notice is provided to the Health Care Financing Administration (HCFA) for its use in notifying all Medicare and Medicaid agencies via its monthly listing (HCFA Publication 69). In order to protect beneficiaries from financial liability, the Medicare contractors notify the beneficiaries when claims are submitted for services rendered by an excluded party. The contractor will pay the first claim submitted by the beneficiary and inform the beneficiary that no more services are reimbursable because of the provider's exclusion status.

We also notify payer agencies administering the Block Grants to States for Social Services (title XX) and Maternal and Child Health Service Block Grants (title V) and send a separate notice to the Federation of State Medical Boards; Office of Civilian Health and Medical Program of the Uniformed Services, Department of Labor, Social Security Administration, Veterans Affairs, and General Services Administration (GSA).

The Federal Debarment List (which precludes excluded providers from participating in Government-wide procurement and non-procurement contracts) is updated through exclusion information that the OIG provides to the GSA. It does not include identification numbers.

The OIG notifies the general public of exclusion actions through the Federal Register which is available in hard copy and through the Internet. In addition, cumulative reports of all exclusions in effect are published approximately twice a year and are routinely released to recipients of the HCFA monthly reports (Publication 69), payer agencies, and on a request-specific basis, to all other interested parties. We remove providers from the cumulative list only if and when they are reinstated. Since its last printing in February 1996, the OIG has distributed more than 750 hard copies and released more than 330 diskettes containing the cumulative sanction report. These copies are in addition to the routine distribution that HCFA makes to all of the Medicare contractors and each of the Medicaid State agencies.

Since early 1996, the cumulative sanction report has been provided on IGnet which is an internet resource of more than 60 Federal Offices of Inspector General. IGnet also gives the public access to the OIG's audit, inspection, semi-annual reports, and other related documents. The user can download the cumulative report as a database file that can be sorted or as a desktop published file that looks like the printed version and is selectively printable. Recently, we added the 'update" exclusion information published monthly in the Federal Register to the same IGnet site. Thus, IGnet contains the names of all of the OIG exclusions currently in effect and is available to anyone with World Wide Web access. Information about accessing this Web page is attached.

Although many users are beginning to go directly to the internet for exclusion data, the OIG also receives and responds to calls originating from the general public, Medicare contractors and State fiscal agents, other Federal and State agencies, credentialing agencies, licensing boards, HMOs, hospitals, and other members of the health care industry. For the first six months of this fiscal year, the OIG responded to 11,317 written requests and 3,640 telephone requests for exclusion information on specific health care providers, mostly medical doctors. We project that more than 25,000 responses to requests will be made before the end of this fiscal year.

There are various other databases and methods for reporting many types of disciplinary or malpractice actions involving a multitude of health care providers. These include the Federation of State Medical Boards Data Bank, the National Practitioner Data Bank, and certain requirements of the Joint Commission on the Accreditation of Healthcare Organizations. The OIG has been working with the Public Health Service and the Health Care Financing Administration to have exclusion data input to the National Practitioner Data Bank so hospitals and licensing boards, in the course of conducting their required responsibilities and routine business, can obtain the current exclusion status of all physicians and dentists in the United States.

Pursuant to the Health Care Quality Improvement Act of 1986, The National Practitioner Data Bank collects information on physicians and dentists concerning malpractice payments, clinical privilege actions, and adverse licensure actions taken by hospitals, insurance companies, licensing boards, and professional societies. This information is then available to all hospitals, licensing boards, and professional societies. If the Medicare provider information is included in the files, OIG sanction information will reach the desired audience and substantially cut down on the number of excluded practitioners who continue to receive inappropriate program payment through hospital cost reports because hospitals are required by law to query all new employees and all current employees on a biannual basis. An interagency agreement is in final clearance, and we expect that the exclusion information will become available to data bank users in Fiscal Year 1997.

While the existing databases are helpful tools, there has been no comprehensive database for the mandatory reporting of "final adverse actions" such as criminal convictions, civil judgements, settlements, administrative exclusions, and disciplinary actions imposed against health care providers.

The new Adverse Action Data Bank to be established under the Health Insurance Portability and Accountability Act of 1996 will facilitate broader communication across the entire spectrum of public and private health care organizations. It authorizes the collection and dissemination of information on any final adverse action taken against any health care provider, supplier, or practitioner. In conjunction with the Department of Justice, the OIG is charged with overseeing this endeavor. We will be a prime contributor to and user of this data bank, while overseeing its structure, procedures, and regulations.

Further, the OIG has been working with the National Registry, which is the HCFA contractor responsible for maintaining the Medicare files on the Unique Physician Identification Number (UPIN), to update its historical exclusion data base to include the UPIN with the subject's personal identifier information. Once assigned, that number is carried on all exclusion notification letters sent to payer agencies and Medicare contractors and is included on all OIG sanction reports. Including these numbers allows the Medicare contractors to more readily identify excluded physicians and lessens the chance that physicians who move from State to State or who use more than one provider number (e.g., group numbers and/or multiple location numbers) can obtain Medicare reimbursement.

We look forward to the day that HCFA assigns unique identification numbers for all health care providers. The availability of such information should make all our jobs easier by broadening the scope of the notification process and by substantially reducing the opportunities for inappropriate program payments and recidivism.

We are convinced that this level of communication has a far-reaching effect on excluded providers. It tells payer agencies that all program reimbursement must cease; it alerts employers that the subject has been shown to be untrustworthy and has a history of disciplinary actions; it puts third party payers and licensing board authorities on notice that a sanction has been imposed and the reasons for it; and, it provides an opportunity for the ongoing exchange of information between Federal, State, and private components dedicated to policing the health care industry. Public Law 104-191 now requires unique numbers for all providers and will allow for a more manageable, efficient, and effective system.

Coordination with the Congress

The OIG testifies before this subcommittee regularly and has made recommendations for the development of a uniform provider agreement, for the use of unique physician identification numbers, and for extending the scope and penalties of the exclusion process itself.

Mr. Chairman, you and Congressman Schiff, your subcommittee, and the full committee supported our proposal to have the Medicare contractors and Medicaid State agencies made liable for and restoring any inappropriately spent program funds that were caused by their failure to implement exclusions timely and accurately. We thank you for that, and we continue to believe that unless these agencies are made financially liable for their mistakes, there is little incentive for doing the job properly. We ask for your continued support in this endeavor.

We are pleased that many of our recommendations on the application of certain health anti-fraud and abuse sanctions have been considered and included in recent statutory changes. Such changes include expanding sanction authorities to cover all Federal health care plans and establishing statutory authority for minimum periods of exclusion for certain individuals and entities subject to permissive exclusion from Medicare and the State health care programs.

Project WEED

Finally, I would like to describe an initiative I mentioned earlier. We developed Project WEED last November to increase the number and quality of exclusion cases being developed by our field offices. After our budget stabilized, we began this endeavor to ensure that we do the best we can with available resources. The project ensures, through staff training and improved guidelines, that the documents and information necessary to process these cases are being gathered and developed in a timely, consistent, and effective manner.

Eight senior program analysts in our investigations field offices are assigned to the project. Sanction training and an overview of the project goals were provided to the analysts in July. During July and August this team identified over 900 potential mandatory sanctions that had not been forwarded to our office. These leads are currently being pursued. Eleven additional personnel are scheduled to receive extensive sanctions training the week of September 9, 1996.

We know that it is important that the OIG have continuity in the exclusion process. It is also important that the States provide the OIG with the information necessary to make an appropriate exclusion decision. We have learned through our exclusion experience that inconsistencies have developed. This information was also documented in the GAO review. Through the Project Weed initiative, we will resolve the inconsistencies by proper and timely OIG staff training. In addition, we are initiating an outreach effort to State Medicaid agencies to ensure that all required information is forwarded to the OIG.

Thanks to the recently enacted Health Insurance Portability and Accountability Act of 1996, we are fully confident about the future. This new law provides additional budget and manpower allocations to the OIG, strengthens our existing exclusion authorities, requires unique provider numbers, and expands our abilities to impact other Federal, State, and local health care programs.

Attached for the record is general information about available sanction authorities and the exclusion process.

Administrative Sanctions
Authorities and General Information

Sanction Authorities

Title XI of the Social Security Act provides a wide range of authorities to exclude individuals and entities from participating in the Medicare, Medicaid, Maternal and Child Health Services Block Grant and Block Grants to States for Social Services programs (titles XVIII, XIX, V and XX of the Act respectively). By exercising the exclusion authorities, the OIG helps fulfill the Secretary's primary obligation to protect the health and safety of patients receiving care as well as to protect the fiscal integrity of the programs.

The Secretary has delegated 42 administrative authorities to the OIG . The most significant in terms of priority and workload are found in section 1128(a) of the Act which sets forth mandated enforcement provisions and are closely allied with the criminal provisions of the law. This section requires the OIG to exclude any individuals or entities for a minimum period of 5 years if they are convicted of a program-related crime or of any type of patient abuse or neglect.

The recently signed Health Insurance Portability and Accountability Act of 1996 (Public Law 104-191) expands this mandatory provision to include all felony convictions related to health care fraud in any program operated or financed by any Federal, State and local government agency or any felony conviction related to controlled substances.

This new law also provided authority to exclude individuals with ownership or control interest in excluded entities. In contrast, sections 1128A and 1128(b) of the Act permit, rather than require, the exclusion of individuals or entities if the OIG determines the action to be warranted. At its discretion, the OIG takes permissive exclusion actions on misdemeanor convictions for non-HHS health care violations like fraud, theft, financial misconduct; for controlled substance violations; for license suspensions and revocations; for sanctions imposed by other health agencies; for the rendering excessive or unnecessary services; and, for entities owned or operated by excluded individuals.

Coupled with our mandatory exclusion authorities are the Civil Monetary Penalty Law (CMPL) provisions which allow the OIG to administratively impose penalties on persons who make false or improper claims for payments under the Medicare, Medicaid, and other State health care programs. In the past we have has the authority to impose a CMP of "not more than $2,000", an assessment of "not more than twice the amount claimed" for each item or service presented as false or improper claims, and impose a permissive exclusion of the provider from program participation.

The Health Insurance Portability and Accountability Act of 1996 extends the current CMP authority to all Federal health care programs and provides for penalties of up to $10,000 per line item or service, three times the amount of each false claim, and $10,000 for each day a prohibited relationship occurs.

Further, the OIG can exclude health care providers and practitioners who have defrauded or abused the programs or its beneficiaries. The OIG may also exclude based on a recommendation received from a peer review organization because an individual or entity failed to meet their legal obligations to provide only care that is medically necessary, meeting professionally recognized standards, and is properly documented. The new law removed an earlier requirement for a finding of unwillingness or inability to comply with the provider's obligations, raised the monetary penalty amount to $10,000 per violation, and established a minimum one-year period of exclusion.

Finally, the OIG can exclude health care providers who have failed to repay or to enter into an agreement to repay a health education assistance loan. These exclusions are mandatory under section 1892, and the OIG couples that mandatory authority with section 1128(b)(14) to ensure that the exclusion extends to the other programs. These exclusions remain in effect until the debts are completely repaid.

In FY 1995, the OIG obtained more than $296 million in civil monetary and false claim act penalties and assessments and implemented 1,478 administrative exclusions. Of these, 504 were section 1128(a) mandatory exclusions, with the remaining 974 resulting from the permissive authorities delegated under the various provisions of section 1128(b) of the Social Security Act.

Despite disruptions in workflow caused by both Federal furloughs during FY 1996, the OIG expects to implement about 1,500 exclusions by the end of this fiscal year. As of July 31, 1996, we had implemented 1,237 exclusions, of which 463 were mandatory and 774 were permissive.

Alternatives to Exclusions

As an alternative to excluding an individual or entity from program participation, the OIG may impose a number of civil monetary penaties for a variety of fraud or abuse violations including fraud, billing or charging violations, patient and beneficiary protection issues, circumvention of regulatory requirements, patient "dumping", physician protection, and improper disclosure of information.

The OIG or Department of Justice may determine that a case cannot be easily prosecuted and that the taxpayers are better served by settling the case rather than expending the OIG's limited resources to further investigate it. When a decision is made to settle a case with a monetary penalty, various safeguards are included in the settlement agreement. Since most of the settlements involve payments over a period of time, the safeguards include not discharging the debt if the individual files for bankruptcy, excluding the individual or entity if they default on the settlement, and recently, if the settlement is with an entity, establishing and maintaining a voluntary compliance program.

Compliance programs are designed to prevent the recurrence of the improper billing practices that prompted the civil monetary penalty settlement. Corporate compliance programs are quite specific in terms of actions a company must take to remain in the Medicare and Medicaid programs. The OIG institutes appropriate safeguards, and sharply reduces the likelihood for continued improper activity before deciding to enter into a compliance agreement, rather than to exclude. Currently, there are approximately 40 to 50 compliance plans in effect; and it is anticipated that, with the tremendous reception that this program has been given by the health care industry, the caseload will more than double in the next fiscal year.

Effect of an Exclusion

Once an exclusion takes effect, program payment may not be made for items or services furnished, ordered, or prescribed by the excluded individual or entity. Additionally, no Federal or State health care program funds can be used to pay any salary or fringe benefits, including administrative or management services, related to the delivery of a health care item or service rendered to a program patient by an excluded individual or entity.

The OIG may exclude any health care entity (such as a hospital or clinical laboratory) if an excluded individual has a direct or indirect ownership or control interest of 5 percent or more in it, or is an officer, director, agent, or managing employee of that entity. This is true whether or not the excluded persons are compensated for their services. Violating this prohibition could result in criminal prosecution by the Department of Justice, and/or the imposition of civil monetary penalties against the excluded individual/entity or the employer by the OIG. (Note: Emergency items or services, under certain conditions, may be paid for by Medicare.)

The exclusion notice to the subject defines the effect of the exclusion and the subject's appeal rights. If the exclusion was taken under the Civil Monetary Penalty Law authorities or because of kickback violations, the excluded party may request a hearing before an Administrative Law Judge (ALJ) and receive a decision before the OIG implements the exclusion. In all other cases, the exclusion is in effect while awaiting the hearing and its outcome. Appeals of ALJ decisions are decided by the Departmental Appeals Board. The subject may then appeal the administrative decision to the district court. Very significantly, less than 0.34 percent of all OIG-implemented exclusions have been reversed on appeal.

The OIG is required to give government-wide effect to all exclusions it imposes. The Federal Acquisition Streamlining Act of 1994 mandates and expands the government-wide effect of all debarments, suspensions, and other exclusionary actions to Federal procurement, as well as non-procurement programs. Thus, all OIG imposed exclusions must be effectuated not only for all Departmental programs, but also for all other Executive Branch procurement and non-procurement programs and activities. This means, for example, that a health care provider excluded from Medicare, Medicaid, and other State health care programs will be unable to continue participating in the Civilian Health and Medical Program of the Uniformed Services (CHAMPUS) program administered by the Department of Defense or in the Federal Employee Health Benefits Program administered by the Office of Personnel Management.

Reinstatement to the Programs

Reinstatement to Medicare, Medicaid, and the other State health care programs is not an automatic process. The exclusion notice issued to a health care provider specifies that, at the conclusion of the period of exclusion, the provider has the right to apply for reinstatement under the provisions of the statute and the regulations.

The OIG will terminate an exclusion and reinstate the provider only if we determine that, during the period of exclusion, the subject has not committed an act for which a civil monetary penalty could be assessed or has not committed an act which would result in an additional exclusion be imposed. Further, the OIG must determine that there are reasonable assurances that the types of actions which caused the original exclusion have not and will not recur.

If the OIG determines that the subject's request for Medicare reinstatement should be approved, we notify the subject and other appropriate parties including the Health Care Financing Administration, Medicare contractors, and the State agencies. The State health care programs may reinstate the subject into their programs upon receipt of the notice from the OIG, unless reinstatement is not available under State law or the State health care program had established a longer period of exclusion under its own authorities and procedures.

Sections of Social Security Act Under Which Exclusions Are Imposed

1128 (a) (1) – Program-related conviction

1128 (a) (2) – Conviction for patient abuse or neglect

*1128 (a) (3) – Felony conviction relating to health care fraud in any Federal/State/local government health care program

*1128 (a) (4) – Felony conviction relating to controlled substance

1128 (b) (1) – Conviction relating to health care fraud (non-HHS)

1128 (b) (2) – Conviction relating to obstruction of an investigation

1128 (b) (3) – Conviction relating to controlled substances

1128 (b) (4) – License revocation or suspension

1128 (b) (5) – Suspension or exclusion under a Federal or State health care program

1128 (b) (6) – [Formerly 1862 (d) (1) (B) and (C)] – Excessive claims or furnishing of unnecessary or substandard items and services

1128 (b) (7) – [Includes former 1862 (d) (1) (A) cases] – Fraud, kickbacks and other prohibited activities

1128 (b) (8) – [Formerly 1128 (b)] – Entities owned or controlled by a sanctioned individual

1128 (b) (9) – Failure to disclose required information

1128 (b) (10) – Failure to supply requested information on subcontractors and suppliers

1128 (b) (11) – Failure to provide payment information

1128 (b) (12) – Failure to grant immediate access

1128 (b) (13) – Failure to take corrective action

1128 (b) (14) – Default on health education loan or scholorship obligations

*1128 (b) (15) – Individuals controlling an excluded entity

1128Aa – [Formerly 1128 (c)] – Imposition of a civil money penalty or assessment

1156 (b) – [Formerly 1160] – PRO recommendation

* Health Insurance Portability and Accountability Act of 1996

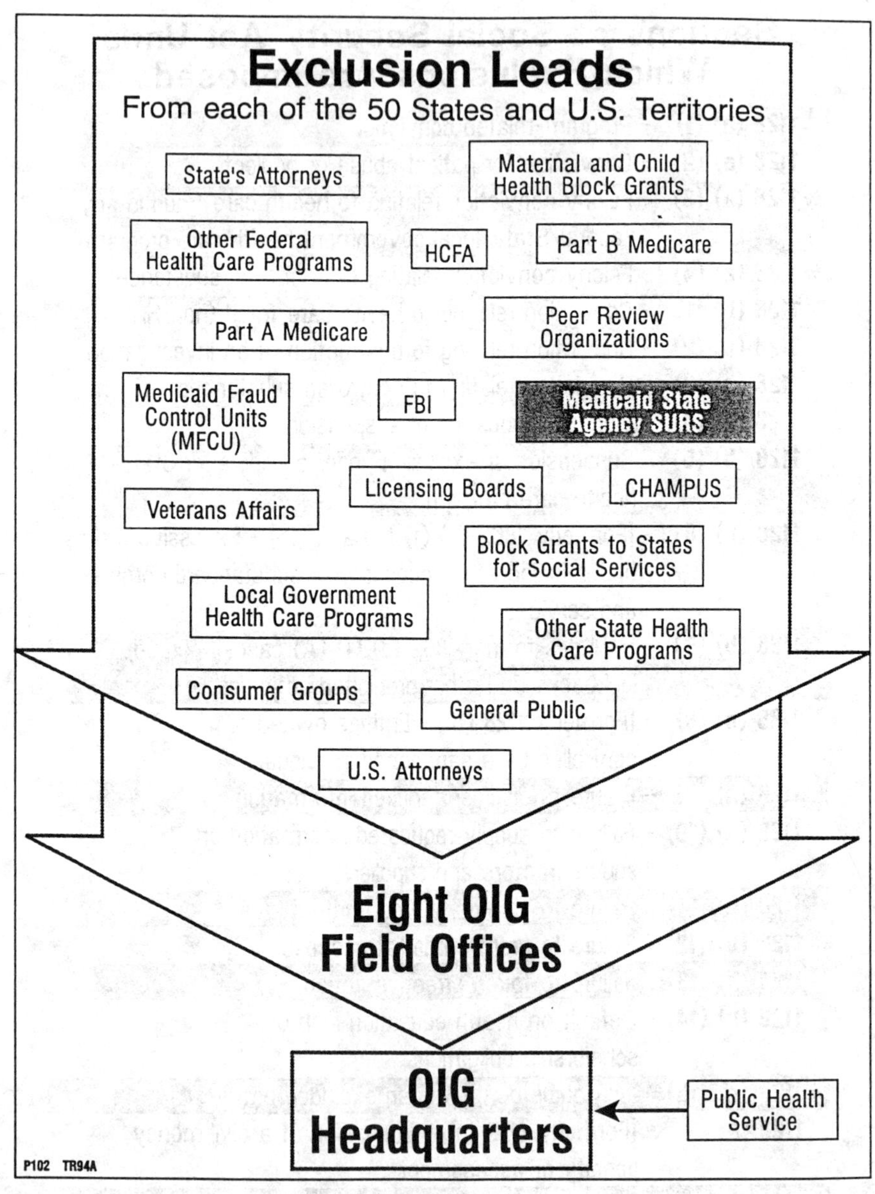
Exclusion Leads
From each of the 50 States and U.S. Territories
State's Attorneys
Maternal and Child Health Block Grants
Other Federal Health Care Programs
HCFA
Part B Medicare
Part A Medicare
Peer Review Organizations
Medicaid Fraud Control Units (MFCU)
FBI
Medicaid State Agency SURS
Licensing Boards
CHAMPUS
Veterans Affairs
Block Grants to States for Social Services
Local Government Health Care Programs
Other State Health Care Programs
Consumer Groups
General Public
U.S. Attorneys
Eight OIG Field Offices
OIG Headquarters
Public Health Service
P102   TR94A

Exclusion Notice Process

Individual Notification Letters[1]	Copies	National Reports
Medicare carrier(s) Medicare intermediary(s) MetraHealth (RRB) Medicaid State agencies Title V State agency Title XX State agency Licensing board(s) Employer, if known	Attorney, if known Public Health Service[2] Department of Justice[2] U.S. Attorney[2] Peer Review Organizations[2] Office of Personnel Management	**MONTHLY** Internet[3] Federal Register HCFA Pub-69 All payor agencies Federation of State Medical Boards Federation of State Podiatric Boards Office of Civilian Health & Medical Program of the Uniformed Services Department of Labor Social Security Admin. Veterans Affairs General Services Admin. (Federal Debarment List) **CUMULATIVE** Internet[3] Monthly recipients Payor agencies Public information on request
cc: HCFA RO		

Abbreviations:
RRB = Railroad Retirement Board
HCFA RO = Health Care Financing Administration Regional Office

Note: Exclusion data will be posted to the National Practitioner Data Bank beginning in FY 1997 and will be posted to the new Adverse Action Data Bank when it becomes operational.

[1] In State(s) where subject known to be.
[2] If appropriate
[3] URL=http://www.sbaonline.sba.gov/ignet/internal/hhs/invlist.htm

Visit the OIG's Exclusion List on the Web . . .

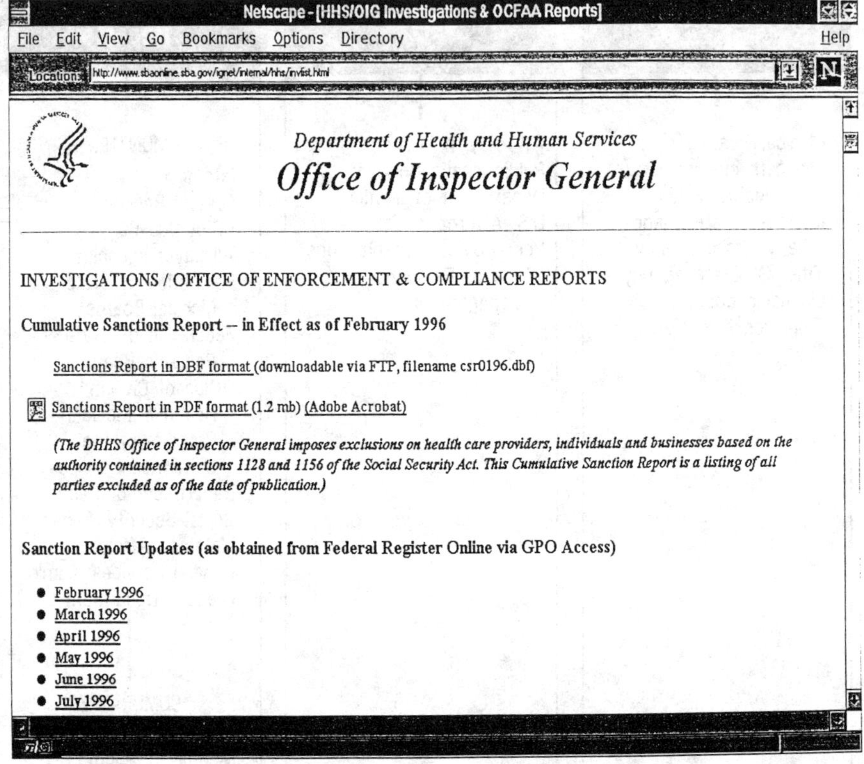

Find us at this World Wide Web address: *http://www.sbaonline.sba.gov/ignet/internal/hhs/invlist.html*

This page is a part of **IGnet**, the internet site of the Inspector General Community.

Department of Health and Human Services
Office of Inspector General

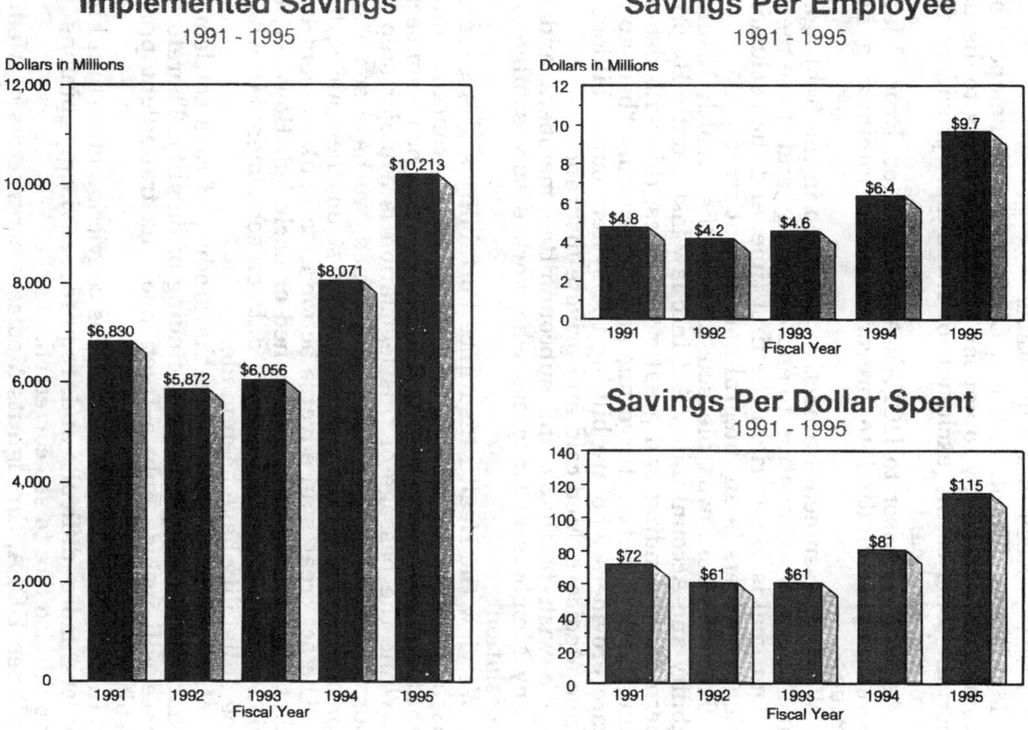

Mr. SHAYS. Thank you. I think we'll go with you, Ms. Berek, and then we'll proceed to ask questions.

Ms. BEREK. Thank you. Mr. Chairman and members of the subcommittee, I'm happy to appear before you today to discuss the important topic of the exclusion of fraudulent providers from Medicare and Medicaid.

As senior advisor to HCFA's Administrator, Bruce Vladeck, I am personally committed to preventing and minimizing health care fraud.

We have assumed a proactive approach in the fight against fraud and abuse by attempting to end costly pay and chase methods.

Our goal is to pay right the first time, and the exclusion of fraudulent providers is an integral part of that strategy.

The President was pleased to sign the Health Insurance Portability and Accountability Act into law last month. By providing for permanent funding and greater penalties, this will also strengthen our hand in better targeting and prosecuting "bad apple" health care providers who are bilking the system out of billions of dollars from Medicare, Medicaid and private insurance.

We wish to thank the subcommittee members and all of the many Members of Congress who worked successfully to pass this legislation.

We view the Health Insurance Portability and Accountability Act as a major breakthrough and note that it contains many of the antifraud provisions that the administration has been seeking.

While the passage of this legislation is a major step forward in our efforts to combat fraud and abuse, we have some suggestions for improvements that would further strengthen our abilities.

The act creates an adverse action data bank to identify providers that have either been sanctioned or excluded. However, this provision prohibits the inclusion of data on settlements in which no finding of liability have been made.

Many adverse actions are the product of case settlements which characteristically include no finding of liability. Therefore, the data base will include only a fraction of the fraudulent providers and will be much less effective.

In addition, the new law makes conviction of certain kinds of providers more difficult and requires advisory opinions which we would also like to see corrected.

When HCFA, through its Medicare contractors or Medicaid State agencies, discovers a potentially fraudulent solution, there are a number of actions that might be taken—prepayment reviews, suspension of payment, denial of payment, or referral to law enforcement authorities and/or recovery of overpayments.

HCFA does not have the authority to remove fraudulent providers from Medicare and Medicaid. It is the HHS Office of the inspector general that has that authority, and HCFA refers cases to the IG for investigation and followup.

Further, we cooperate with other law enforcement agencies, such as the Medicaid Fraud Control Units, the Department of Justice, the FBI, and U.S. attorney's offices.

Once a provider has been excluded from Medicare or Medicaid, the OIG informs us. We inform our contractors, the State agencies and other State licensure agencies.

All Medicare claims processes in States are expected to ensure that excluded providers are not paid.

One of HCFA's most promising initiatives in assisting in both the detection of early action against fraudulent providers and in helping with exclusion is the Fraud Investigation Data Base or what we call the FID.

It is a Medicare case tracking system. Medicaid State agencies and Medicaid Fraud Control Units now have access to the system, and we are planning to add Medicaid data as well.

The FID disseminates information to and from law enforcement agencies, Medicare, Medicaid agencies and contractors regarding exclusion as well as identifying ongoing cases so that, in fact, the payers will know that another payer is looking at this provider while they're being looked at.

One of the more difficult problems in achieving coordination of excluded providers has been the lack of unique identifiers for each provider.

Following two pilot efforts and after extensive national consultation with other public and private payers, HCFA is currently leading a joint Federal/State initiative to establish and maintain a comprehensive system of unique provider identifiers.

In the past, the issuance of billing numbers has been independently done by each payer. Under the National Provider Identification System, one number, the NPI, will be used for all Medicare billing and, hopefully, with the recent health care reform legislation, all payers, and that should improve the initiative. The use of the National Provider Identification System will identify those providers who have been excluded from Medicare.

Further, as Medicaid and other Government programs adopt the NPI, providers will no longer be able to hide their exclusion or other adverse action from one program to another.

HCFA is in the process of developing a Medicare information system which will, among other things, assist in our provider exclusion.

MTS has been designed to consolidate all Medicare processing, fee-for-service and managed care into one standardized system. We plan to use MTS to identify and review aberrant billing patterns and to prevent inappropriate payments.

MTS will also provide us with an enhanced ability to keep out fraudulent providers. The MTS is designed to use the National Provider Identifier, which will flag excluded providers and those identified as potentially fraudulent.

This data base will be accessed before the claim is paid, and, if appropriate, the payment will be suspended or denied.

HCFA is also in the process of implementing improved provider enrollment procedures. The best way to fight fraud is to allow only honest players in the game. By improving the provider enrollment process and raising the standards for both participation in both Medicare and Medicaid, HCFA will be able to prevent fraudulent providers from coming in in the first place.

I'd like to tell you about another piece of legislation that we are hopeful will aid us in our efforts to prevent fraudulent providers from enrolling in the Medicare Program.

This past April, the President signed into law the Omnibus Consolidated Recisions and Appropriation Act. This included a provision known as the Debt Collection Act. This provision is intended to facilitate collections by Federal Government and streamline procedures. The act permits HCFA to require its providers to supply us with their Taxpayer Identification Number when submitting an application to enroll in Medicare.

This will help us to track providers even if they change their names and addresses. However, because the Taxpayer Identification Number cannot be traced to the Social Security number for providers who incorporate or who are employees of other providers, we believe that additional legislation that would allow us to collect Social Security numbers directly would be helpful.

As a further tool, HCFA will be adding exclusion information of excluded health care providers to the National Practitioner Data Bank.

This data bank now contains all malpractice information as well as licensure and clinical privilege actions.

The NPDB assists State licensing boards, hospitals, and managed care organizations in conducting investigations of the qualifications of practitioners they seek to license, hire or grant clinical privileges to.

Including exclusion information in the NPDB will prevent prohibited employment agreements and inappropriate Medicare/Medicaid payments.

I could not testify without mentioning Operation Restore Trust. HCFA, the OIG and the Administration on Aging have formed a partnership with Federal and State law enforcement agencies.

This partnership has been aggressively cracking down on Medicare and Medicaid fraud and abuse. The ORT demonstration in five States together account for 40 percent of Medicare and Medicaid beneficiaries. As you know, they're New York, Florida, Illinois, Texas, and California.

In Florida, the Medicaid agency and the National Supplier Clearinghouse have developed a successful program to allow enrollment of only qualified DME dealers.

The State Medicaid agency has taken the initiative—and I'm really sorry Rufus will not be here—to require surety bonding for providers at several categories, including durable medical equipment.

And as part of this partnership, HCFA is going to, on a demonstration basis, move to requiring surety bonding for DME dealers in Florida because it has been so successful.

ORT's success is due largely to coordination among the agencies involved on the State and Federal level during investigations before cases are even ready for exclusionary action.

It is our plan to assure that this approach expands on a State-by-State basis so that we can continue in the process.

HCFA, in the Medicaid Program, has recently established a Medicaid fraud and abuse network involving all of our regional offices to serve as a forum for coordinating antifraud activities.

We have also established a Medicaid council that provides an exchange of ideas between the State SURS units as well as the Medicaid fraud control units and HCFA, the IG's office and the FBI.

In conclusion, as we enter the 21st century, HCFA is actively improving its use and availability of computer technology as well as coordination with other entities to keep pace with the rapid change occurring in the health field.

Advanced information technology is essential to preventing fraud and abuse. We are also forging new partnerships to increase cooperation among Federal agencies, State entities, and private insurance to protect the Medicare and Medicaid programs from fraud.

We look forward to working with the subcommittee and other Members of Congress in this fight. Thank you.

[The prepared statement of Ms. Berek follows:]

INTRODUCTION

Mr. Chairman and members of the Subcommittee, it is a pleasure to appear before you today to discuss the very important topic of the exclusion of fraudulent providers from Medicare and Medicaid. We are seriously committed to acting aggressively to respond against all forms of fraud, waste and abuse. Excluding fraudulent providers is essential in protecting the Treasury, the Medicare Trust Funds, the state governments, and the beneficiaries.

As Senior Advisor to HCFA's Administrator, I am personally committed to controlling and minimizing health care fraud and have the full support of HCFA's Administrator Bruce Vladeck in my anti-fraud efforts. We have assumed a pro-active approach in the fight against fraud and abuse by attempting to end costly pay and chase methods. Our goal is to pay right the first time. The exclusion of fraudulent providers is an integral part of HCFA's strategy.

Health Insurance Portability and Accountability Act of 1996 (P. L. 104 - 191)

The President was pleased to sign the Health Insurance Portability and Accountibility Act into law last month. In enacting this legislation, we have acheived a long-overdue victory in ensuring that workers who change their jobs can keep their health insurance. By providing for permanent funding and greater penalties, this law also strengthened our hands in better targeting and prosecuting "bad apple" health care providers who are bilking the system of billions of dollars from Medicare, Medicaid and private insurance. We wish to thank Subcommittee members and all of the many members of Congress who worked to successfully pass this legislation.

The new health insurance law creates the Health Care Fraud and Abuse Control Program to be coordinated by HCFA, OIG, and the Attorney General. The program, which will fight fraud in Medicare, Medicaid and private health plans, is funded by mandatory appropriations from the Medicare Hospital Insurance Trust Fund and the general fund of the Treasury. Under the auspices of the Control Program, HHS will have the resources to implement the lessons learned from Operation Restore Trust nationwide. Building upon the successes of the five-state demonstration project, HCFA will be able to coordinate with the OIG, the state agencies, as well as law enforcement to fight fraud in both Medicare and Medicaid, and to ensure that a provider that defrauds one program is not able to defraud the other.

The new health insurance law also adds new mandatory exclusions from Medicare and Medicaid for felony convictions related to health care fraud or controlled substances. It allows the Secretary to exclude providers convicted of misdemeanors related to health care fraud from the Medicare and Medicaid programs for a minimum of three years. It also adds new permissive exclusions from Medicare and Medicaid for individuals whose health care licenses have been revoked or suspended, or for individuals controlling a sanctioned entity. Further, where a practitioner has failed to successfully complete a Peer Review Organization corrective action plan, or has grossly failed to meet quality standards, the Secretary may exclude them from Medicare for a minimum of one year.

The new law also expands all Medicare and Medicaid criminal provisions to all federal health programs and establishes new civil money penalties and extends many current Medicaid and Medicare civil money penalties to all federal health care programs, except OPM sponsored plans.

We view the Health Insurance Portability and Accountability Act of 1996 as a major breakthrough, and note that it contains many of the anti-fraud provisions that the Administration has been seeking. The Congressional Budget Office conservatively estimates that these provisins will save over $3 billion. So, while the passage of this legislation is a major step forward in our efforts to combat fraud and abuse, we have some suggestions for improvement that would further strengthen our abilities.

Recommendations for Improvement

The Act creates the Adverse Action Data Base to identify providers that have either been sanctioned or excluded, i.e. those providers that have been subject to a final adverse action. However, the provision prohibits the inclusion of data on "settlements in which no findings of liability have been made." Many final adverse actions are the product of settlements of cases, and characteristically, no findings of liability are made. This provision may encourage many other providers that would currently admit liability to challenge HHS's determinations of their behavior with the goal of entering into a settlement which avoids being listed in the data bank. If significantly larger number of providers do this, the data bank will then list only a fraction of fraudulent providers thereby becoming much less effective. The President's bill did not exclude final adverse actions resulting from settlements, providing the Administration with comprehensive data on adverse actions.

Second, the new law weakens the penalties for fraudulent claims. Under the new law, the government now has to prove that providers acted with "deliberate ignorance" or "reckless disregard." Previously, we could levy penalties on providers for submitting fraudulent claims if we could prove that they "should have known" the claim was fraudulent.

Third, the new law, unlike the President's bill, requires advisory opinions. The OIG has stated that advisory opinions on intent-based statutes (such as the anti-kickback statute) are impractical if not impossible. Because of the inherently subjective, factual nature of intent, it would be impossible for HHS to determine intent based solely upon a written submission from the requestor.

PROGRESS

While passage of this legislation gave us greater tools in our fight against fraud and abuse, this administration did not wait for legislation to aggressively attack fraud and abuse in the Medicare and Medicaid programs.

Until several years ago, there was little coordination between Medicare, Medicaid, the enforcement agencies, and other entities interested in curbing health care fraud and abuse. However, I am pleased to report that now significant progress is being made in our war on fraud and abuse. During this Administration, HCFA has substantially increased its efforts, forged new partnerships, and developed new strategies to ensure the integrity of the Medicare and Medicaid programs. HCFA has pioneered fraud and abuse initiatives and financed state-of-the-art information technologies to detect and deter fraud and abuse. Although we still face significant challenges and have much work before us, we are achieving many successes in our efforts to strengthen, preserve, and protect the Medicare and Medicaid programs.

Excluding providers is a major tool by which we protect the Medicare and Medicaid programs. Therefore, I would like to explain the process by which a provider or supplier is excluded.

PROVIDER EXCLUSION PROCESS

When HCFA discovers a potentially fraudulent situation, it takes immediate action to protect the Medicare Trust Fund and the beneficiary by suspending or denying payment and recovering overpayments. HCFA does not have independent authority to remove fraudulent or abusive providers from the Medicare or Medicaid programs. It is the HHS-Office of the Inspector General (OIG) that has this authority to impose exclusions. HCFA refers cases to the OIG and assists in the investigations. Further, we cooperate with other enforcement agencies such as the Medicaid Fraud Control Units, the Department of Justice, the Federal Bureau of Investigation, and the U.S. Attorney's office.

Once a provider has been excluded from either Medicare or Medicaid, the OIG informs HCFA, its contractors, state Medicaid and licensure agencies, and others. The OIG also publishes a list of excluded providers quarterly in the *Federal Register* as well as on the Internet. All Medicare claims processors and states work to ensure that providers being paid or applying for billing numbers are not currently under an exclusion.

HCFA is currently using technology in new ways as well as strengthening the enrollment process so that excluded providers remain excluded and do not attempt to re-enter Medicare or Medicaid by moving to a new state or setting up a new business under a new provider or tax identification number.

EXCLUSION TOOLS and INITIATIVES

1. Fraud Investigation Database (FID)

One of HCFA's most promising initiatives in assisting in the exclusion of fraudulent providers is the Fraud Investigation Database (FID). We began implementing the FID in May, and expect to have complete up-to-date information by December. The FID is a case-tracking system to record and disseminate information regarding exclusions. It will contain extensive national Medicare and Medicaid fraud data as well as comprehensive information on all excluded providers. The FID is intended to assist HCFA and our partners in the identification of excluded providers as well as those who are allegedly defrauding the programs. For example, a Medicare contractor in one area can use this information to ensure that the providers it is reimbursing have not been excluded through the actions of another contractor.

In an effort to enhance coordination of the exclusion process, the FID is also accessible to the Medicaid anti-fraud agencies such as the Medicaid Fraud Control Units and the Surveillance and Utilization Review Systems. We expect to soon be able to obtain data from these Medicaid entities on cases and information related to the providers that they suspect to be fraudulent.

The FID is also designed to ensure the coordination of anti-fraud activities undertaken by our law enforcement partners and to facilitate the monitoring of cases referred to the OIG, the FBI or the U.S. Attorneys. We are pleased to report that several other federal government entities, including the OIGs of the Postal Service, Office of Personnel Management, and the Department of Labor, are in the process of acquiring access to the FID. It is our goal to make sure that a provider who defrauds Medicare or Medicaid cannot defraud other federal programs.

2. <u>National Provider Identifier System</u>

HCFA is currently leading a joint federal and state initiative to establish and maintain a comprehensive, unified system of provider identifiers. This system will build upon the success we have achieved in the issuance of unique billing numbers for medical equipment suppliers. With unique provider identifiers, we will have the enhanced ability to verify information for each provider seeking to bill Medicare. In the past, this verification and the issuance of billing numbers have been independently done by each of the 70 Medicare contractors, leading to different numbering methodologies and an inability to create a central Medicare database for the verification of provider eligibility. In general, a provider will have only one billing number, regardless of the number of Medicare contractors that it bills. Under the National Provider Identifier System, one number (i.e. the National Provider Identifier - NPI) can be used for ALL Medicare billing.

The use of the National Provider Identifier System will help to ensure that only legitimate health care providers are enrolled in the Medicare program. This will occur through the identification of providers that have been excluded from Medicare reimbursement. Further, as Medicaid and other government programs adopt the NPIs, providers can no longer hide from their Medicare exclusions and other adverse actions through the use of a separate Medicaid or other federal health care program number.

The Health Insurance Portability and Accountability Act of 1996, which I will discuss later, expands upon HCFA's efforts to create a standard system of provider billing numbers, by requiring the Secretary of HHS to adopt standards for providing a unique identifier for every provider for all health care programs. We are in the process of making sure that the requirements of this Act are consistent with our plans to have the National Provider Identifier System operational. We are also working to encourage states, private payers, and other Federal agencies to adopt the NPIs.

3. How the Medicare Transaction System Will Assist in Fraud Detection and Provider Exclusion

HCFA is in the process of developing an automated Medicare claims processing and information system, which will, among other things, assist in our provider exclusion efforts. The Medicare Transaction System (MTS) has been designed to consolidate the currently fragmented Medicare claims processing into one standardized system. MTS will greatly improve HCFA's ability to profile data on a national or regional basis by type of service. We plan to use these profiles to identify and review aberrant billing patterns and to prevent inappropriate claims from being paid in the first place, thus avoiding the need to chase down those fraudulent claims that have already been paid. The MTS will integrate data from Medicare Part A, Part B, and managed care and provide the opportunity to build on best practices in information systems and to incorporate new technology to facilitate innovative investigative techniques.

One of the many benefits of the MTS will be its enhanced ability to keep out fraudulent providers. The MTS is designed to use the National Provider Identifier System. This system, as I mentioned previously, will be a record of all providers and suppliers who are certified to bill Medicare for medical services or equipment provided to our beneficiaries. If a provider is excluded from the Medicare program, or has been identified as fraudulent, that provider will be flagged in the database. This database will be accessed before the claim is paid.

The MTS will improve our ability to coordinate claims processing with medical and fraud review. When a bill or claim is entered into the MTS from an excluded provider or supplier, payment will be denied. Additionally, the OIG can levy a civil monetary penalty on any excluded provider who continues to bill Medicare or Medicaid. We have a civil monetary penalty case tracking system, which will use the claim submission information from MTS to assist in identifying excluded providers and ensuring that they do not continue to bill.

4. The National Supplier Clearinghouse

HCFA established the National Supplier Clearinghouse (NSC) to enroll suppliers of durable medical equipment and supplies in Medicare. The NSC verifies supplier data on all applications and matches suppliers, owners, and managing employees listed on new applications to a file of all equipment suppliers to ensure that there has been no previous history of fraudulent or abusive practices by any of the listed individuals. If a previous history is noted, the application is denied.

The NSC also verifies that medical equipment suppliers meet Medicare standards. If the NSC determines that the standards are not met, then it will not issue a Medicare billing number. Further, any supplier found to be out of compliance with these standards will have its Medicare billing number revoked. Additionally, there is a re-enrollment process every three years, which prohibits suppliers no longer in compliance with standards to retain their Medicare billing numbers and provides the NSC with updated information. The NSC has recently revoked approximately 1,300 supplier numbers during the latest round of re-enrollment.

The NSC is also investigating oxygen licensure requirements. This would help to ensure that a supplier is legitimate before claims for oxygen or related services are paid by Medicare. As a result of this effort, the NSC has revoked almost 600 oxygen supplier numbers for improper, invalid, non-existent, or otherwise incorrect licensure information.

To date, we believe that the NSC system has saved the Medicare program millions of dollars and was instrumental in our response to fraud in the South Florida area which I will address shortly.

5. New Enrollment Process

Presently, HCFA is very limited in its ability to deny providers entry into the program and, more importantly, to make the Medicare provider enrollment process a fraud and abuse prevention tool. We are in the process of using our administrative authority to expand our efforts at preventing fraudulent providers from continuing to bill Medicare.

We are currently drafting a regulation that would establish new standards for all entities and individuals billing Medicare and make it more difficult to abuse the use of a Medicare billing number. This will help to ensure that legitimate information will not be used by fraudulent suppliers to obtain Medicare billing numbers, thereby protecting both the beneficiary and the legitimate billers from fraudulent and unprincipled billers. We hope to publish the proposed regulation for public comment within one year.

HCFA is also implementing improved, standard Medicare provider and supplier enrollment procedures which increase the standards for enrollment in the Medicare program. And, for the first time, all Medicare contractors will use the same provider enrollment form. I am pleased to report that in April, HCFA received approval from the Office of Management and Budget to use the new Medicare Provider/Supplier Enrollment application for providers and suppliers not certified through state survey and certification procedures.

I'd like to tell you about another piece of legislation that we are hopeful will aid us in our efforts to prevent fraudulent providers from enrolling in the Medicare program. This past April, President Clinton signed into law the Omnibus Consolidated Rescissions and Appropriations Act of 1996, which includes a provision known as the Debt Collection Improvement Act. The Debt Collection Improvement Act is intended to facilitate collections by the federal government and encourage the coordination of information within and among federal agencies and streamline procedures. This Act permits HCFA to require that its providers and suppliers indicate their tax identification number (TIN) when submitting a Medicare enrollment application. The TIN for an individual is the person's Social Security Number (SSN). This will allow us to track providers through a unique personal identifier even if they change their names or addresses. However, because the TIN cannot be traced to the SSN for providers who incorporate or who are employees of other providers, we believe that additional legislation that would allow us to collect Social Security Numbers directly would be helpful.

The best way to fight fraud is to allow only honest players into the game. By improving the provider enrollment process and raising the standards for participation in both Medicare and Medicaid, HCFA hopes to avoid fraud in the first place.

6. Boston Provider Exclusion Project

HCFA's Boston regional office is currently conducting a review of state policy and procedures involving excluded Medicaid providers in Massachusetts. This review is designed to identify the best practices and make recommendations to other regions about provider exclusion practices that they use. HCFA believes that the Boston review may prove to have national applicability, and we will encourage other regions to conduct similar reviews.

7. National Practitioner Data Bank

In addition to the above mentioned tools, HCFA is facilitating the dissemination of information on physicians and other licensed health care providers concerning malpractice payments, licensure actions, and clinical privilege actions through the National Practitioner Data Bank (NPDB) which is maintained by the Public Health Service. The NPDB assists state licensing boards, hospitals and managed care organizations in conducting investigations of the qualifications of the health care practitioners they seek to license, to hire, or to whom they wish to grant membership or clinical privileges. To perform a thorough investigation of a practitioner's qualifications, these entities also need to know whether or not a practitioner has been excluded from Medicare or Medicaid. HCFA is entering into an agreement with the Public Health Service, whereby we will provide a list of excluded providers to be posted on the NPDB. Having the NPDB identify excluded providers will help to prevent prohibited employment arrangements as well as inappropriate Medicare and Medicaid payments. Further, it will reduce the level of effort and redundancy for both the health care industry and the federal government by having the NPDB distribute the exclusion reports to authorized health care entities in addition to their own reports.

ADDITIONAL ANTI-FRAUD INITIATIVES

1. The South Florida Task Force

As I mentioned earlier, the NSC's monitoring system became instrumental in HCFA's response to fraud in the South Florida area. South Florida has consistently proven to be a problem area for health care fraud.

In 1994, HCFA launched a task force to attack fraud and abuse in South Florida. Medicare contractors, Medicaid state agencies, U.S. Attorneys, and Medicaid Fraud Control Units worked together to detect fraudulent billing practices in Medicare and Medicaid. In one of the joint activities, the group matched Medicare and Medicaid data, thereby making it easier to identify patterns of aberrant billing. For instance, when the South Florida task force identified medical equipment suppliers as a source of fraud, HCFA met with the NSC, the Medicare contractor, the Florida Medicaid program, and the Florida state licensing agency to obtain their input in developing improved supplier applications.

Building on the success of the South Florida Task Force, similar workgroups have now formed in a dozen states. Further, HCFA also opened an office in Miami in September 1995, to focus on minimizing fraud and abuse. This office supports the investigative and law enforcement efforts of several of our partners, including the FBI, the U.S. Attorney's office, and the contractors. It also conducts outreach and educational activities. The NSC is also establishing on-site representation in the South Florida area to conduct extensive site visits of Medicare supplier billing number applicants to ensure legitimacy.

2. Operation Restore Trust

Based upon HCFA's successful experience in South Florida, the Secretary launched a two-year demonstration in which HCFA, the OIG, and the Administration on Aging formed a partnership with federal and state law enforcement agencies. This partnership, known as Operation Restore Trust (ORT), has been aggressively cracking down on Medicare and Medicaid fraud and abuse. The ORT demonstration targets the five states which together account for 40 percent of all Medicare and Medicaid beneficiaries -- New York, Florida, Illinois, Texas, and California.

With a first-year budget of about $4 million dollars, ORT has identified approximately $39 million dollars that should be returned to the Medicare Trust funds due to restitutions, settlements and recovery of overpayments.

3. Attacking Medicaid Fraud

The Medicaid programs are run by the states, with guidance and technical assistance from HCFA. HCFA's role in attacking Medicaid fraud is therefore primarily to provide resources and technical assistance that facilitates the exchange of information.

In recent years, HCFA has devoted greater attention to cooperating with states and other entities to attack Medicaid fraud and abuse. HCFA is providing increased technical assistance and encouragement for Medicaid anti-fraud programs. We are working to improve the exchange of information between Medicare and the nation's 54 Medicaid programs, including federal and state law enforcement agencies. Since states administer Medicaid, states cooperate with Medicaid Fraud Control Units, which are federal-state funded entities devoted to investigate Medicaid fraud. The OIG, FBI, U.S. Attorney, and state Attorney Generals are also involved in Medicaid investigation and prosecution.

<u>Medicaid Fraud and Abuse Network</u>

In conjunction with Medicaid anti-fraud efforts, HCFA has recently established the Medicaid Fraud and Abuse Network which is comprised of employees from HCFA's central and regional offices. This Medicaid Network serves as a forum to coordinate anti-fraud activities, provide an information clearinghouse, and initiate Medicaid anti-fraud prevention projects. HCFA also has developed partnerships with states' Surveillance and Utilization Review Systems (SURs) Units and states' Medicaid Fraud Control Units (MFCUs) to facilitate the detection, referral, and ultimate prosecution of Medicaid fraud and abuse cases.

<u>Medicaid Fraud and Abuse Coordinating Council</u>

As a result of the SURs/MFCUs joint effort, HCFA has established the Medicaid Fraud and Abuse Coordinating Council (Medicaid Council). It provides a forum to exchange ideas; to discuss and resolve problems which may arise between SURs and MFCUs; and to sponsor workshops, conferences, and seminars involving anti-fraud issues.

HCFA is currently conducting training sessions sponsored by the Medicaid Council to ensure that all states, along with the OIG and the FBI, have an opportunity to participate in anti-fraud managed care workshops. National associations on behalf of SURs and MFCUs have also agreed to jointly develop a cross-training program designed to enhance their communications and to ensure that the two entities work together more closely.

CONCLUSION

Since Medicare and Medicaid first began three decades ago, millions of Americans have been helped in paying their medical bills. It is most appropriate that as the 30th Anniversary of Medicare and Medicaid is celebrated, HCFA is even more committed to ensuring that 70 million of our most vulnerable Americans continue to have access to high quality and cost-effective health care. HCFA is committed to act aggressively to pursue all forms of waste, fraud, and abuse.

As we enter the 21st century, HCFA is actively transforming its computer technology to keep pace with the many rapid changes occurring in the health care field. The implementation of information technology is essential in combating and preventing fraud and abuse. Further, we are forging new partnerships to increase cooperation among the federal agencies, state entities, and private industry, to protect the Medicare and Medicaid programs from fraud, waste, and abuse. HCFA and I look forward to working with this Subcommittee and other interested members of Congress in implementing its health care fraud and abuse initiatives.

Mr. SHAYS. I thank you for your statements, both of your statements. They were helpful to the committee, and we, likewise, look forward to working with both of you.

At this time I'd call on Mr. Souder to ask any questions.

Mr. SOUDER. I was reviewing some of the list of some of the people who have been disqualified, and maybe, Ms. Brown, you can address this question.

It looks like most of them are individuals. Is there anything that keeps an individual from forming a separate entity that deals just with Medicaid or Medicare?

In other words, if you were, like, a doctor, form a name of a company that then would provide the services?

Ms. BROWN. Well, we have certainly found that many of the more egregious offenders, those that are really professional crooks, are very adept at applying for a right to bill Medicare under some different entity name.

In fact, Judy Berek showed me an announcement very recently of a company that we were just getting out of the system who put out an announcement saying, "We're doing business. We're expanding. Only the name has changed. All the people are the same."

Of course, we immediately took action against the new entity as well, but this was something they sent to all their clients in order to convince them to continue doing business with them even though they were one of those that had committed offenses.

Mr. SOUDER. In just reviewing the list, it looks like many of them are potentially small abusers, and you probably have some that are huge abusers. Is that true?

Ms. BROWN. That's true.

Mr. SOUDER. Is it the typical 5 percent do 90 percent of the damage, or is it less?

Ms. BROWN. As a percentage, I can't give it to you. But of course, there are many individuals who are getting convicted. Then we take the exclusion action against them.

Larger companies aren't as often convicted, but then, there are many individuals involved when they are. That's because it often is only one portion of the company, rather than the entire entity that is responsible for the offense. We're very careful about putting companies out of business unless the whole company looks as if it is responsible for the kinds of offenses that are going on.

Sometimes we work out something where a company divests itself of those portions of the company where the offenses had occurred. Then those individuals responsible for the offenses may be excluded.

Mr. SOUDER. Has there ever been any sampling or maybe the field people what happens to the people on that list after they get listed? Do many of them go out of business?

Ms. BROWN. I think that's true. Certainly, the excluded companies can no longer operate, and our exclusion extends to all Government health care programs.

So when they lose the ability to take care of CHAMPUS patients, as well as anyone under Medicare or Medicaid, it usually puts them out of business.

Those exclusions are also for a set period of time, unless the court makes it a permanent exclusion. So once these people have served that time or they have cleared up the problem that got them on the list, they can apply for reinstatement.

We do have some continuing dialog with these folks, once they apply. If they have met the criteria, then they're taken off the exclusion list.

Mr. SOUDER. Do you have, I assume, some sort of a prioritization process by how many dollars there were, the severity of the crime as far as whether you track them closely to see if there is any suspicion, if they reappear similarly?

When you're filtering through all those different groups that come in, are you matching to see the size of it so you can make sure the resources are there, plus, if you see it pop up from, say, three or four different places, do you prioritize in that way?

Ms. BROWN. We do prioritize; and, of course, that's part of the problem. We're questioning whether the priority is right.

It's partly a resource problem, but we try to do those things that would get the most egregious offenders out of the program—those that have mandatory exclusions.

You know, if the process were simply a matter of reporting and forwarding information, it would be very easy to fix.

But, in fact, we have to accumulate a lot of information, including the sentencing, which may come long after the conviction, because that would be a consideration as to the length of the exclusion.

We have to look at the egregiousness of the offense. We have to gather a lot of information and have all of it available before a decision can be made.

Also, we have to provide notice back to the people so that they can have 30 days to respond to us and let us know of any mitigating circumstances which might influence either the length of time of the exclusion or whether or not they should be excluded, if it's a permissive exclusion.

All of those things are done before the package is sent on to headquarters. Once it comes to headquarters, it takes probably, on average, about a month to process.

It might go 2 months, but not longer than that, assuming all the documentation is together at that point.

So there is a lot of work that goes into these, particularly the permissive exclusions, because we have to justify the action. It's a pretty drastic action for the person who ends up excluded.

Ms. BEREK. Can I add something on the individuals? One of the reasons that we think getting Social Security numbers on all providers or suppliers is important is because that is the unique identifier everyone has, and we can track them.

We have a demonstration going on now in Mr. Shays' home State actually where we are going through all of the individuals who have been excluded—cooperatively with the FBI, because they have access to Social Security numbers—and matching it with the employment and payroll records of all health care providers in the State who employ individuals to see how many of those individuals have, unbeknownst to any of us, gone to work for another provider.

These are the individuals who don't bill directly, pharmacists, nurses, and so on. But that is the reason why Social Security numbers make such a difference.

And we hope, in this demonstration in Connecticut, to be able to get some idea of the scope of the problem there.

Mr. SHAYS. The gentleman is allowed to continue, but would you forward the results of that to the committee? I think that would be very interesting.

Ms. BEREK. Absolutely. We'll be happy to set up a briefing for you on it as well.

Mr. SHAYS. That would be great. Mr. Souder.

Mr. SOUDER. I wanted to ask one additional question, if I could, of Ms. Berek. When you raised a question that I had alluded to earlier—I've referred to it in things pending—you have in which no findings, like the podiatrist we heard about earlier.

Given the fact if many of these people no longer are in business and it hasn't been established clearly in a court their conviction, is there any way that any kind of a list could be made of people who used to be doing business who are no longer doing business without a judgmental statement on it, just saying that they've withdrawn from the program, an interim?

Because I think many people, then, could have a warning signal also could make an independent judgment; in other words, may make a decision.

What I find is that, in Fort Wayne, the word of mouth on doctors is fairly strong and pharmacies and others that if so and so ever came in and was drunk, well, they did a surgery or that type of thing, it moves through the community pretty fast.

Now, maybe it's different in Chicago or a bigger city, but at least in a mid-size and certainly in small towns, that's going to be somewhat true.

At the same time they may find that that has changed or it was an unusual incident, and it's worth the risk, but some sort of a thing, because we also know that there are a lot of complaints filed that indeed don't necessarily have merit.

And enough people are getting familiar enough with our legal system that they don't necessarily presume somebody is guilty, like we used to, in a higher percentage of the cases?

Is there something, a transition other than just implying that the person's guilty and that somehow they have a mark on their head when, in fact, we haven't proven it?

Ms. BEREK. That is the purpose of the FID. The reason we designed that system was so that when a contractor now, which would be a Medicare payer, thinks they have enough evidence of fraud to refer a case to the inspector general's office, they enter everything they know about that situation into the data base.

Every other Medicare contractor has access to that, every other payer who pays for Medicare, and we are now in the process of enrolling Medicaid, SURS units, and Medicaid Fraud Control Units.

And we have had requests from Postal Service, FBI, various other groups that investigate health care fraud, in addition to the inspector general's office, to get access to the data base, and we are enrolling them in it.

Mr. SOUDER. Even if there is no liability?

Ms. BEREK. Right. Well, no. If we refer it to the inspector general, there would be—this is from the contract with the inspector general. So there would be a financial liability involved in those cases.

And it is that data base which will serve for us, ending with not just the final action but the beginning action. And that would allow, for example, if a doctor is billing for patients—and I'll give you the most—durable medical equipment, take that, is billing for patients in Florida, because the bills must track to, with DME, the location of the beneficiary, those bills would be paid by our DMERK in South Carolina.

If the DME company is selling DME for a person in Pennsylvania, that bill would be paid by our contractor in Connecticut, because that's who pays the DME claim, that person.

Well, if there is a problem with a provider, now, with the FID, there is a system where each contractor can look in and see, "He's got something on that guy. I've got something on that guy."

And you know either to put together material to pursue a larger case, or you know to begin to watch, which I think is what you're asking us to do, and say:

Now, wait a second. Maybe this provider needs to be put on prepay review for every claim. Maybe this provider needs to have their payment suspended because it appears from this settlement they owe Medicaid $1 million. Why is Medicare paying them anything?

And that's part of what the Debt Collection Act also wants us to do. So that system is designed for that purpose, and we think that it will make a huge difference.

It is new. It has been up and running since the summer. We are enrolling people in it. We are putting back cases into the system now, but we think it will do that and get to the biggest piece of this, which is the financial fraud.

Mr. SOUDER. Thank you.

Mr. SHAYS. Thank you. Mr. Towns.

Mr. TOWNS. Thank you, Mr. Chairman. Let me ask, you made a statement, and I wasn't sure what you meant. You talked about the reduction in staff.

Ms. BROWN. Yes, sir.

Mr. TOWNS. When did this happen?

Ms. BROWN. Well, we have had regular reductions in staff since 1992, and last year we lost about 800 more people and $10 million.

Now, the new law, Public Law 104–191, Kennedy-Kassebaum, will give us some stabilized funding and allow us to increase our resources.

And that should help considerably to allow us to pursue the kinds of fraud that we are aware of and also do some aggressive work where we feel there are probably problems.

Mr. SHAYS. If the gentleman would yield 1 second, it would be helpful to the committee to understand you really have two functions.

You're like the Labor inspector general. You have an operational function besides an investigative one.

So when you talk about, say, the reduction of staff, what the bill does is give you staff for this particular area, correct?

Ms. BROWN. No, sir. We have audit, investigative, and analytical work, as well as this exclusion and civil monetary penalty function.

Mr. SHAYS. But the inspector general also looks at programs of HHS.

Ms. BROWN. Yes. We may audit them, or we look at them for waste of different types.

Mr. SHAYS. And the bill is going to allow you to use your resources in the whole area?

Ms. BROWN. Just for health care waste, fraud, and abuse.

Mr. SHAYS. Right.

Ms. BROWN. So it would depend. And of course, since the money is coming out of the Medicare trust fund, we intend to use the additional resources for Medicare fraud to improve the Medicare programs, because that nexus with the funding we feel is very important.

Mr. TOWNS. Would the gentleman yield?

Mr. SHAYS. Yes. You have the floor. Thank you.

Mr. TOWNS. Not Medicaid? Just Medicare?

Ms. BROWN. There is a great deal of overlap between the two, and we have other funding as well. So we will continue to pursue Medicaid; and we will, of course, be pursuing anything in Medicare that is overlapping.

These offenders do not confine themselves to one program. We usually find that it's not only Medicare-Medicaid but also CHAMPUS and even other Government health care programs.

We've returned money to all of those funds, when we get a conviction or a settlement with one of these offenders.

Mr. TOWNS. When I look at this, I look at it in two ways. I think that we could be a lot more aggressive in dealing with the Medicare situation, in terms of numbers, than Medicaid.

When we talk about it, I know sometimes we, sort of, mix both of them up, but the point is that I think that Medicare is something that we could move a lot more aggressively on in terms of dealing with the fraud and abuse problem.

Let me just, sort of, go back to the restore trust operation. I'm anxious and eager to see in terms of what comes out of that, but I must say that I have some real concerns because of some things that are happening within the industry.

I come from a tristate area in terms of Connecticut, New Jersey, New York. At one point you had facilities within the State would merge, but now you have facilities merging across State lines.

I'm not sure how you can deal with that, because you could have a company in New York actually working in Connecticut, a company in Connecticut actually working in New York.

And I'm not sure in terms of how we deal with this under the present structure, in terms of restore trust.

Ms. BEREK. I'll talk about the billing end of it, and I will yield to the inspector general to talk about the investigating end of it.

One of the reasons we need MTS is because right now all contractors operate and do payment on a State-by-State basis, and, in fact, some kinds of providers have the right to elect a contractor to pay their bills and a fiscal intermediary that can be on the other side of the country, if they choose.

And that's the way the law is structured, so that's what we now do. Under MTS, what we will be able to do is, although people may bill through an agent in a particular location, all the bills will be centrally processed.

And so people won't be able to, sort of, you know, bill Illinois 1 week and Pennsylvania the next to try to get away from us.

But for those providers now that operate across State lines, if they are operating honestly, they should have selected a contractor that pays them no matter where they are located, unless they are a DME provider.

And that's because we felt this was the best way to clean up DME that we've done it differently, and the contractors pay whether the claim is New York, New Jersey, Connecticut.

There will be one fiscal intermediary that will be paying the bill for that hospital or nursing home operation.

Mr. TOWNS. That's Medicare.

Ms. BEREK. That's Medicare. On Medicaid, they will bill on a State-by-State basis, and they would have to have a billing number with each of the State Medicaid agencies, which is one of the things that will help us enormously in the implementation of the Kennedy-Kassebaum bill.

We are now putting up this national provider identifier system, which, under the current rules, is voluntary for anybody but Medicare, although we have indications that the States Medicaid programs are interested in participating, and CHAMPUS is interested in participating, and these groups have been working with us.

But under the new legislation, if the Secretary designates the NPI and it meets the standards of the legislation, then we would have one provider number nationally for every payment system for every provider. So it would help us enormously with that problem.

Mr. TOWNS. Yes. Ms. Brown.

Ms. BROWN. Our authority, of course, crosses State lines.

Mr. TOWNS. Right.

Ms. BROWN. This is good because most of the crime does too. Operation Restore Trust was a demonstration project where we tried to put concentrated resources in five representative States.

However, when we find something going on in any one of the five and it overlaps into other jurisdictions nearby, we continue with that investigation.

We don't say that we can only look at what occurred within that State. It's just that that's where the concentrated effort and additional resources were put in.

We wanted to demonstrate how much we could accomplish if funding were given to us. If you would put up that other chart.

I might say I have been inspector general in five major agencies, including Department of Defense, and I have also been a military inspector general.

I have never run into problems such as are true in HHS, and that is with the amount of fraud that we're talking about. Now, even though our resources have been cut, I want to show you the way our recoveries have occurred.

Last year, 1995, we brought back $10.2 billion—that was just my office—with things that we started. Now, some of those are program changes, legislative changes and so on, and those are evaluated by what the Congressional Budget Office uses as the figures.

But $10.2 billion, that is, on average, with every person on the staff, including clerical help and others who don't get involved in these things, that averages $9.7 million per person, and $115 for each dollar spent.

So you can see that our priorities, we have had to weigh them very, very carefully and try to do what was best for the program, which would bring back the most money, stop the most egregious offenses.

Certainly, I have a lot of crime that I am well aware of through the input to our office that we have not been able to get to.

Now, the new funding will help us tremendously, but I want to explain that we know we are not doing everything that ought to be done and that the kind of recoveries that are coming in not only show that we're somewhat efficient, which I'd like to show, but it also shows the extent of the problems and what it is we're dealing with here.

So all of these things, including the tremendous effort that HCFA has made—because we have worked together closely, and there wasn't something in the position that Judy Berek now occupies.

This is a new initiative that they started to have somebody that is looking at program integrity and who works very closely with our office.

And we have joined efforts so they've put in a lot of new controls and tracking systems, and we are benefiting from that because we are able to get the information that they're accumulating. We're working together very closely to improve these programs.

I would like to add one thing, because you have concentrated on it during this hearing, and that is the unique identification number.

Having worked in the agencies I have, which includes Social Security, Department of Defense, I have never seen a large system, and I was in development of——

Mr. SHAYS. Never seen a what system?

Ms. BROWN. I have never seen a major system before that didn't have some kind of unique identifier for everybody in that system.

I don't know how anybody could create a system like Medicare and Medicaid where there is no unique identifier. We have Social Security numbers, but we're not allowed to use them for most purposes.

We can't print them on the list that's available to the public and available to those other than the payors. We're not even allowed to have access to them for some purposes.

We cannot get a system with high integrity if we don't absolutely insist on having a unique identifier for everybody who is able to get payments out of that system.

The confusion with names and things is something that just exists, and we have to be very careful.

Until now, we have had no unique identifiers. We're going to spend a tremendous amount of money trying to put them in.

Or maybe Congress will allow us to use Social Security numbers or something like that that could be a unique identifier that already exists and that we can track back.

When there is an entity, we can see who the individuals are that they employ or who manage that entity as well as the individuals who bill us as individuals.

When we get somebody with a unique identifier out of the system, it will be very easy for everybody to implement those actions into their systems.

Mr. TOWNS. Well, let me just, very quickly clarify a point, Mr. Chairman, if you would allow me.

Mr. SHAYS. That's all right. You have the floor.

Mr. TOWNS. This is a very complicated issue. I agree with you. I think that we have to do something. I mean, there is no question about that.

I think when we talk about it in terms of quality of care. We're also talking about the abuse factor of from a financial standpoint where people are just taking the money from the Government and sticking it in their pockets.

I think somewhere along the line we have to make certain that there is enough staff around to really address this issue, if we're serious about fraud and abuse. I think that's one issue.

The other thing—I guess this question would be for you, Inspector—could you describe the forms in which the exclusion lists is transmitted to HCFA, what form, is the information transmitted to HCFA? And is HCFA capable of receiving it?

Ms. BROWN. We provide that to HCFA in electronic form, and we also provide them a hard copy. They can use the electronic submission to update their existing files without having to re-enter all of that data. And they also have a hard copy, for immediate reference, should they need it.

Mr. TOWNS. Let me just ask, I guess to HCFA, please describe how you distribute the OIG exclusion information nationwide. How do you get this information out?

Ms. BEREK. It's distributed electronically to the contractors. Every 1 of the 70 contractors in the 54-State Medicaid agencies get that information from us both on paper and electronically.

And once we put it in this National Practitioner Data Bank, we think it will be much more accessible because it's a bank that people have to go to for other things.

I mean, for example, we expect a managed care plan not to have an excluded provider as part of that managed care plan.

And they are using that data bank now to see whether or not the provider has been sanctioned in any other way other than for financial fraud through us.

So by putting this in the same data bank, we think that in terms of employment, already excluded providers, we will get a much higher rate of obedience, whatever, accuracy.

Mr. TOWNS. Conformity. Let me ask this question, because you're here to educate us as well.

Do all of the States have compatible data systems that would be able to receive this information and be able to make use of it?

Ms. BEREK. No, they do not. Each State Medicaid agency has its own data system, and they are not necessarily compatible.

And, in fact, our 70 contractors use multiple data systems that are not compatible now, which is why we need to put up MTS so that all the Medicare data will be on one compatible system. So that will allow us to do things on a prepay basis, because we will be able to do it quickly.

We will be able to both pay at the speed of light and get the exclusion and all that other information in there so that it can be matched prior to payment electronically.

At this point, we are working to build compatibility with State Medicaid systems in various locations. It's one of the things that's going on in the five States where we are trying to combine and merge data.

One of the obstacles to the compatibility of information is the fact that we use different identifier numbers to pay, and so that that is a huge obstacle to leap, in terms of getting toward compatible data systems.

Inspector General Brown has some staff in Texas that has tried to merge, for people in nursing homes, all of the Medicare and Medicaid data, and they are just beginning to use it.

And it took us almost 8 months just to build the data base that would have all of the Medicare payment data, all of the Medicaid payment data from all parts of the program, and they're now using it. So it is still a very difficult thing to do.

Ms. BROWN. But there are no unique numbers to identify this. Even with wonderful technology, we can't merge data without unique identifiers. We are very, very limited as to what we can do.

Ms. BEREK. What we had to do in Texas is focus it not on the providers but on the beneficiary because, from the Medicare view, the beneficiary has one number, if it hasn't been bought or sold by one or stolen.

And so we had to actually focus on the beneficiary's number as the way we gathered all the information in.

Mr. SHAYS. You give me a good seguay to invite the gentleman from Texas to ask questions.

Mr. GREEN. I apologize. I was talking about another issue that you brought up, and I know the Texas example. But let me first, Ms. Berek, I know you mentioned the MTS system, but in this committee, we held hearings on Medicare fraud, and this is Medicaid.

So even with the MTS system in place—and that's why I wanted to ask you where we're at on the schedule for the MTS. But again, that won't help us with the Medicaid, because the States are the contractors.

Ms. BEREK. It will help with Medicaid in one piece. If we are all working off the same provider or supplier number, it will make an enormous difference.

In order for MTS to go up, we must move to the National Provider Identifier system. We must have one set of numbers for the providers in Medicare.

As I say, we have had cooperation from Medicaid agencies and other insurers that they would participate. Now you've given us the legal authority to say they must participate.

So I think it will help. So I think MTS will help in Medicaid as well because of the enumeration, the accurate enumeration of providers. I am not the manager of the MTS implementation.

Mr. SHAYS. Thank God, huh?

Ms. BEREK. I don't know if you're saying that it means that if I was the manager, it will be in terrible shape.

Mr. SHAYS. No, no, no. That's not what I mean.

Ms. BEREK. Am I supposed to be insulted?

Mr. SHAYS. No, no. You do not need to be insulted. You just should be grateful you're not in charge.

Ms. BEREK. I'm willing to admit I'm grateful I'm not. The pieces of it that I focus on is what impact will it have on program integrity issues and how we put up the provider enumeration system, because I believe that that is one of the keys to it.

And I can tell you that as they are putting it up, they are putting as the first two priorities putting managed care in—because there is no real managed care data system in place at this point—and in building the pieces that have to be built to do the program integrity activities to begin to unify them.

So those are the priorities of putting this system up right now as we, sort of, plan for the conversion.

I do know enough to tell you that we are in the final stage of negotiations for the platform, and until those negotiations are finished and we have a contract and a plan, it will be very difficult to answer the question.

I will ask the folks putting it up to give you the answers to those questions as soon as we complete these negotiations and have them.

Mr. GREEN. I'd like to have that, Mr. Chairman, because as you recall, the GAO told us the MTS system was at risk.

Mr. SHAYS. Yes.

Mr. GREEN. Let me go back to some questions, particularly the use of Social Security numbers.

Ms. BEREK. Yes, sir.

Mr. GREEN. If a business provides, approves a contract and they send a check to someone, they have to have some type of employer ID number. We don't do that with Medicaid providers?

Because I mean, if you send a check out to some provider, you don't have their Social Security number, their employer ID number or something or their tax number?

Ms. BROWN. There are many different types of numbers in the system, and one provider can have a dozen different numbers very easily.

Mr. GREEN. What does the IRS use? Because I know somehow they can access—if you received 1,000 checks in a given year and it's using their same——

Ms. BEREK. They can link the taxpayer ID number or the employer ID number to the Social Security number, and we can't.

So that somebody could ask IRS for 50 taxpayer ID numbers and then come to us with 50 different taxpayer ID numbers to get 50 different Medicare or Medicaid numbers.

Mr. GREEN. OK.

Ms. BEREK. And we can't link back and find out that that's all one person, and that's the difference in terms of what Social Security numbers will give us.

Mr. GREEN. We've also noticed—and I was surprised, Mr. Chairman, that there was an article a year ago—I have some folks in my own district who have three or four Social Security numbers.

I never realized people except by mistake may have applied, but that is a problem that we have. And again, even using Social Security numbers may not be——

Ms. BEREK. Three or four is better than 50.

Mr. SHAYS. That's true.

Mr. GREEN. It depends on the district. I was interested in my colleague from New York's question about the States and their compatible data systems.

On Medicaid—and again, coming from Texas and the need that you have—how can we require that data systems at least match?

Because again, what we're seeing is more decisions being pushed down to the State, and frankly, a lot of times they make the ultimate decision on what computer they're buying or what system they're buying.

But also can't we require them to, whatever they can buy, at least be able to match with the Federal system?

Ms. BEREK. One of the things I said earlier was when we were putting up the provider identification system, the NPI, we had the cooperation of States and the interest of States who participated.

It is in the States' interest to participate in that system and build the compatibility. In Operation Restore Trust, most of the States have been absolutely cooperative in everything we have done and shared information and data and worked to build the compatibility.

So I think as all of us are seeing the value of having the data compatible and having the provider numbers be the same, I hope we will not have to mandate onto the States that they do this, but I think it will be something that we will be able to move forward.

In our dealings with the Medicaid programs at this point, we see the interest in that kind of cooperation, and we now are looking at, when we approve new systems going up—Texas is, in fact, in the process of putting up a new Medicaid system that is a fraud detection system.

HCFA, in the old days, would just approve a State system going up and not think about whether it was compatible with the Medicare system or how information can be shared, and that doesn't happen anymore.

If we're going to pay 90 percent for the development of a system, we want to make certain that that system will be compatible.

And so that is happening. So I would like to hope that we would be able to do it without having to come to you and say make the States do this.

Mr. GREEN. Mr. Chairman, with your permission, Ms. Brown, let me ask one question about that GAO identified OIG's problem with the area of different offices have different criteria.

And again, if we expect the 50 States to be compatible, then we really ought to expect our offices to be able to work with each other, and if you could just address the OIG findings on that.

Ms. BROWN. Yes. It isn't that they have different criteria. We all use the same OIG manual; and they have an agent's handbook; and it has all of the criteria in there and so on. What they have is different priorities.

So it depends upon the workload in those different offices how much time they can devote to this effort.

So there is some of them, for instance, that would say if somebody isn't excluded for over a year, and another one might say 2 years. That is, from the State program or the conviction or whatever it was would not last longer than that, they wouldn't process that because they felt that we would get very little time on the exclusion list for the time that it took to get it in.

And there wasn't enough time to do everything, and that would include, of course, the other investigative work that an office is doing.

So some offices are very shorthanded and have a lot of very high priority work. Others might have a little less, or they might have some trainees in that office that could devote a little more time to this effort.

There was inconsistency in the way field offices handled things but not in the rules, requirements, enforcement, or what it was they were supposed to put together in order to send cases to headquarters.

Mr. GREEN. And Mr. Chairman, my last. On your charts you brought up there about the implemented savings and the savings for an employer for the dollar spent, when I was in the legislature, we would always, when we had to have a certified number for our budget, we could always go to our State controller and say, "OK. If we gave you 100 new auditors, what could you certify as our available revenue?" And they would do just what you're doing here.

I'm sure the IRS does that with the Appropriations Committee or the subcommittee, just like Ways and Means may.

And you have done that with this, that if we gave you another 100 employees to look for fraud, you could get us $115 back for every dollar we spend on those investigators. Is that correct?

Ms. BROWN. I think there will be a diminishing return because we are, of course, cherry-picking. We're taking those things that are going to be the biggest payoffs——

Mr. GREEN. Largest and most egregious.

Ms. BROWN. We went through an awfully lot of this effort both with congressional staff, and with OMB in determination for more resources under Kassebaum-Kennedy and the President's MAP program and so on.

There were various proposals to get us more resources and they came up with slightly different figures and different things, but we all agreed that there was a tremendous payback. They did decide that the resources were worthwhile.

And I think they are using something like a 7 to 1 return. As long as we are returning 7 to 1, they ought to be financing this effort. Of course, there is also a tremendous deterrent effect with effective enforcement.

Mr. GREEN. And that 7–1, is that agreed to by both the OMB and the Congressional Budget Office?

Ms. BROWN. That's what they would be looking for with the new resources.

Mr. GREEN. And that's both agencies?

Ms. BROWN. Yes.

Mr. GREEN. Thank you, Mr. Chairman.

[The prepared statement of Hon. Gene Green follows:]

Statement of Representative Gene Green
.bcommittee on Human Resources and Intergovernmental Relations
September 5, 1996

Thank you, Mr. Chairman. I am pleased that this subcommittee is continuing its series of hearings on waste, fraud, and abuse in the Medicare and Medicaid programs. In past hearings, we have learned of the difficulties in removing fraudulent providers from the national health care programs, even the difficulties in charging them with a specific health care crime. From this we included a fraud provision in the recently passed Kassebaum-Kennedy health care bill and I want to complement the Chairman, Mr. Schiff, and my ranking member Mr. Towns for their work on this issue over the past two Congresses.

During today's hearing, I would like to explore with the witnesses how this law will be implemented and how we can continue to reduce waste, fraud and abuse in our health care system.

Mr. SHAYS. Thank you. What I'd like to do, I just have a few follow-up questions. I'd like to invite Ms. Aronovitz to come up, if you have any comment that you'd like to make in response to what you've heard.

You, kind of, perked up once or twice, so please feel free to just come back. You're more than welcome to. Please have a seat.

All three of you have been very helpful to this committee. We had the GAO make a suggestion, three suggestions, that would get the States to weed through exclusion referrals and make sure that the most serious are properly documented and sent to the OIG region.

And then the second was get the OIG to fast-track referral some States that meet mandatory exclusion criteria and get them to the OIG headquarters for action.

And third was to get the OIG exclusion lists more easily accessible and more widely available. Were those, basically, the three points?

Ms. ARONOVITZ. Right.

Mr. SHAYS. Would either of you like to add to that list or focus on a different area?

Ms. BEREK. I think I would focus on getting a unique provider supplier identifier, because that will make the systems work.

I mean, one of the reasons it's hard to do is that the provider does not necessarily have the same identifying number between programs or between——

Mr. SHAYS. I think you've documented that. But I just want to know that would be your highest priority?

Ms. BEREK. That's my highest priority.

Mr. SHAYS. I was going to say that's what it would be, but I wanted you to say it as your highest priority. Yes.

Ms. BROWN. I think unique provider numbers are needed for all aspects of managing these systems effectively. And certainly, getting rid of a lot of the fraud in the systems is the most critical problem.

Mr. SHAYS. Just refresh my sense of why we exclude Social Security. I know it's a privacy issue, but it has become such an absurdity because you have to write it on checks sometimes.

You have to write it down so many times, and I'm tempted to say it's none of your business just because I'm tempted to say it. But, basically, anybody who wants to get a Social Security number ultimately can get it.

Ms. BEREK. Except Government agencies.

Mr. SHAYS. Except the Government, except the people who have to pay out the money. Would your recommendation be that we just use the Social Security list?

Ms. BEREK. I don't know whether we would want to necessarily use the Social Security list because, for example, a hospital is a provider. And whose personal Social Security number would you use?

Mr. SHAYS. Right.

Ms. BEREK. So that it is not necessarily, for all instances, the number of choice. But yes, I want the Social Security numbers of the principals who own that hospital or manage that hospital, because if a doctor is excluded for nefarious behavior, I don't want him to be able to run a hospital.

And if all I'm looking at is the employer ID number for that hospital, then I have a problem. So I think it may be a mistake to make the Social Security number have to be the identifier, but I think we have to have access to it to match to the identifier so we're sure who the individuals are.

Mr. SHAYS. Do you want a followup question?

Mr. SOUDER. I had a specific question on that from one that came up earlier, too. And that is that one of the problems, if you put the Social Security numbers in for everybody in the group, like a hospital, how would you protect people who may have worked at a place that has been labeled——

Ms. BEREK. We're talking principle. Nobody is looking to get the Social Security number on a routine basis for every employer of every institution.

If there is a problem, you would want to do a match, but what we're looking at in terms of a hospital or a nursing home are a home health agency or a durable medical equipment company is that the people who own 5 percent or more of the interest or who are principal managers of those companies would give us their Social Security numbers.

And if somebody was a principal manager of National Medical Enterprises, I would want to know if they opened up a new business.

They weren't excluded. They're still in the program. But I would certainly want to monitor any institution that one of those individuals was now involved in managing.

And because I can't track that, I can't monitor that. And that's part of when we say we want to, sort of, end pay and chase, if I know somebody who wasn't excluded but makes me a little nervous is in the program, I can watch them up front and not ever have to give something to June Brown, because I can see up front very quickly that there are problems, stop paying them and end it right there.

Ms. BROWN. That is the company we collected $379 million back from.

Mr. SHAYS. So obviously, one issue would just be the unique provider number, and that really was the purpose of putting it in the legislation was to give you that authority.

And now the question is how does that actually get implemented. I'm just trying to see parallels between Medicare and Medicaid.

In Medicare, you have 70 contractors, basically, that you negotiate with. In Medicaid, in a sense, the States become the contractor? OK.

And do you have the authority now with Medicaid to be able to treat them as a contractor like you do in Medicare?

Ms. BEREK. Yes. With the new system, we will be able to say to everybody—I mean, what Congress has mandated the Secretary to do is to establish a single number issuance system that all payers will use, and Medicaid is one of those payers. So that as the system goes up, Medicaid will be mandated to use that number.

Mr. SHAYS. So you treat them, in a sense, as a contractor?

Ms. BEREK. As a contractor, but it also includes private insurance. It just doesn't include Government payers. So it will be Medicaid. It will be CHAMPUS. It will be private insurance.

Mr. SHAYS. This was a recommendation that you all made to us last year, and that didn't make it in the Medicare bill reform and Medicaid bill that we passed and was vetoed by the President.

And that's why we took particular satisfaction—not only did we make it an all-payer, but one simple effort, to me, can be so beneficial.

And you all should know that all three of you were instrumental in that being in the legislation by your speaking out about it.

The other issue is when someone is, basically, going to be on the exclusion list, they drop out before they're going to be on the list.

It just means they're not on the list. So they, then, they could apply for a new number—that's the problem.

I wouldn't want to be on that list. The amazing thing is we just got this off the Internet. I mean, it's a book. I mean, we printed this up.

I wouldn't want to be on this list. I'd be fearful that I might be. I'd voluntarily drop out of the system for a while, and then I'd just reappear. Is that the basic concern?

Ms. BROWN. The offense might be one where we would have permissive exclusion authority, or something like that, but we never even get notice.

They make the agreement with whatever State agency they're talking to. And they'll say, "We'll just not bill you anymore." They back out. We never even know of it or even have the option of considering an exclusion.

Mr. SHAYS. It seems to me anybody with any brains would realize that they're going to be excluded would be wise to just voluntarily drop out and just, kind of, keep a low profile for a while. Yes.

Ms. ARONOVITZ. I should just add that in States that are very aggressive in getting into these voluntary agreements, they make very strict and very complete agreements with people in terms of managing their involvement in the State Medicaid program.

It's not that they disappear for a while and then could just come back. I mean, the States, as far as we could tell, like New York——

Mr. SHAYS. Yes. But they may show up in Medicare.

Ms. ARONOVITZ. Exactly. Exactly. They do an excellent job in getting them out of Medicaid and keeping them out of Medicaid for sometimes extended periods of time.

Mr. SHAYS. In their State.

Ms. ARONOVITZ. But you're right. They do not normally then get referred to either a State licensing board or the OIG. So therefore, they are only excluded from that one program.

Mr. SHAYS. OK. I'm going to finish my questioning. I just wanted to know, do you have any other comment from the GAO? All right.

You did nod your head a few times when both of them spoke while you were up at the table, and that reaffirmed their points, too. So that was helpful. Does any other Member have a question, followup?

[No response.]

Mr. SHAYS. We thank all three of you, and we appreciate all your good work.

We will now go to our third and final panel, consisting of James White, the director of program integrity, New York Department of Social Services; and also Dr. Warren Koontz, Board of Medicine, State of Virginia.

And we were to have a third person, Rufus Noble, from Florida, whose testimony we've put into the record. Thank you both for being here. Remain standing so I can swear you in.

[Witnesses sworn.]

Mr. SHAYS. You might pull your chairs in a little bit closer. It would be a little more friendly here. Thanks. That's great.

Well, it's wonderful to have you both here. I appreciate you waiting. In your testimony, you're more than welcome to do a little ad lib and make reference to what we've already asked.

I think you have a pretty good sense of what our questions are. You may decide you want to focus us somewhere else as well, but the point is feel free to refer to what has happened before. I'll start, I guess, in the order I called you. Mr. White from New York.

STATEMENTS OF JAMES WHITE, DIRECTOR, PROGRAM INTEGRITY, NEW YORK DEPARTMENT OF SOCIAL SERVICES; AND WARREN KOONTZ, BOARD OF MEDICINE, STATE OF VIRGINIA

Mr. WHITE. Mr. Chairman, members of the subcommittee, I'm pleased to be here today to discuss the procedures used to exclude health care providers who abuse the Medicaid Program.

With the cost of health care continuing to grow, it's important that we look at all ways to ensure fiscal integrity.

In New York, Governor Pataki recently established a joint task force on health care insurance fraud to create an interdepartmental approach to identifying and prosecuting individuals involved in this type of activity.

With Medicaid expenditures surpassing $20 billion annually in New York, fighting fraud, abuse and waste has been given new emphasis by the administration in order to do as much as possible to ensure that these expenditures serve their intended purpose of providing care to the needy of our society.

The State Department of Social Services has had the responsibility for Medicaid provider oversight to include auditing, investigating and, when appropriate, sanctioning providers.

The staff responsible for this activity is composed of medical professionals, investigators as well as auditors. And the department works closely with other State licensing and oversight agencies such as the Department of Health and Human Services and the Department of Education as well as the Medicaid Fraud Control Unit.

Over the past several years, New York has certainly had its share of Medicaid fraud. One of the more notable were the lab blood scams, the Medicaid mill problem and drug diversion.

These scams have been well documented and the subject of numerous national media stories. The department learned the value of being able to react swiftly and a need to have regulatory capacity to deal with the scenarios we encounter.

In the administrative arena, we want to be able to move as swiftly as possible to stop the bleeding by cutting off an individual's ability to be paid my Medicaid for services or goods that were provided or ordered which were excessive, not medically necessary or, in fact, fraudulent.

Parts 515 and 504 of the department regulations govern our activities and we believe allow us to aggressively deal with problematic providers.

But this has been an evolutionary process. As loopholes were discovered, administrators took steps to amend existing regulations to deal with each situation.

For example, excluded physicians who have been unable to receive payment for Medicaid were nevertheless able to continue to write prescriptions and orders for medically unnecessary items.

Labs, pharmacies, and durable medical equipment suppliers would fill the orders and claim they were entitled to reimbursement because they had no knowledge that the physician had been excluded.

Our regulations were amended to clearly State that exclusion includes prohibiting reimbursement for any items ordered or prescribed by an excluded physician.

We have also expanded our regulations to allow the department to sanction individuals affiliated with excluded providers, such as owners, lab medical directors, and supervising pharmacists who have had knowledge of or participated in the conduct of the unacceptable practice.

New York notifies HHS–IG and numerous health insurance carriers of all of our exclusion activity.

While strengthening our provider sanctions was a major step forward, we still needed additional ways to deal with the problems we faced.

The department addressed this need by also strengthening our provider enrollment provisions. Part 504 of our regulations defines an important concept; that is, the contractual nature of the relationship between Medicaid providers and the Medicaid Program.

At one point, Medicaid was looked on as an entitlement program for providers in New York. That's no longer the case.

Enrollment applications require more information, get more extensive review and, in many cases, are denied when they're not in compliance with the requirements set forth in part 504.

The department believes that this has prevented many problematic providers the opportunity to defraud Medicaid.

Part 504 also allows the department the ability to terminate its contractual relationship with providers within 30 days upon written notice and without cause.

However, in utilizing this provision, the department has chosen to present providers with the reasons for its decision to terminate. An administrative hearing is not required or provided.

Providers terminated using this mechanism cannot be paid by Medicaid but are not subject to other restrictions. Employment of these regulations has been vigorously contested, but the department has been extremely successful, and landmark case law has been made in cases which have reached the U.S. Court of Appeals.

In New York, providers do have the ability to voluntarily withdraw from Medicaid. This is not a tool that we often utilize, nor do we permit it in situations that we feel are particularly egregious.

It's most likely to occur after the final determination to exclude the provider has already been made and the department and the provider have reached the administrative hearing stage.

If a problem arises with the presentation of the department's case, it may be decided accepting the provider's voluntary withdrawal may be the best resolution.

In conclusion, I would like to say that, in New York, we have implemented regulations that allow us to stop the bleeding while still recognizing provider's rights to due process.

However, we believe that administrators must build the regulatory capability to quickly move against problem providers.

And it is also important, as certainly highlighted this morning, that State Medicaid agencies, and fraud control units and HHS–IG have on-line access to a national data base of provider activity.

Mr. Chairman, this concludes my remarks. I'll be pleased to answer any questions.

[The prepared statement of Mr. White follows:]

Mr. Chairman and Members of the Subcommittee:

I am pleased to be here today to discuss the procedures used to exclude health care providers who abuse the Medicaid Program. With the cost of health care continuing to grow its important that we look at all ways to insure fiscal integrity. In New York Governor Pataki recently established a Joint Task Force on Health Care Insurance Fraud to create an interdepartmental approach to identifying and prosecuting individuals involved in this type of activity. With Medicaid expenditures surpassing $20 billion annually in New York, fighting fraud, abuse and waste in the program has been given new emphasis by the administration in order to do as much as possible to insure that these expenditures serve their intended purpose of providing care to the needy of our society.

The State Department of Social Services has had the responsibility for Medicaid provider oversight to include auditing, investigating and when appropriate sanctioning providers. The staff responsible for this activity is comprised of medical professionals and investigators as well as auditors. The Department works closely with other state oversight and licensing agencies such as the Departments of Health and Education as well as the Medicaid Fraud Control Unit in the Attorney General's Office.

Over the past several years, New York has certainly had its share of Medicaid fraud activity. Among the most notable were the lab blood scams, the Medicaid mill problem and drug diversion. These scans have been well documented and the subject of numerous national media stories. The Department learned the value of being able to react swiftly and the need to have the regulatory capacity to deal with the scenarios we encounter.

In the administrative arena, we want to be able to move as swiftly as possible to "stop the bleeding" by cutting off an individual's ability to be paid by Medicaid for services or goods that were provided or ordered which were excessive, not medically necessary or in fact fraudulent. Parts 515 and 504 of the Department's regulations govern our activities and we believe allow us to aggressively deal with problematic providers. But this has been an evolutionary process. As loopholes were discovered, administrators took steps to amend existing regulations to deal with each situation.

For example, excluded physicians who had been unable to receive payment from Medicaid, were nevertheless able to continue to write prescriptions and orders for medically unnecessary items. Labs, pharmacies and durable medical equipment suppliers would fill the orders and claim they were entitled to reimbursement because they had no knowledge that the physician was excluded. Our regulations were amended to clearly state that exclusion <u>includes</u> prohibiting reimbursement for any items ordered or prescribed by an excluded physician. We have also expanded our regulations to allow the Department to sanction individuals affiliated with excluded providers such as owners, lab medical directors and supervising pharmacists who had knowledge of or participated in the conduct of the unacceptable practice. New York notifies HHS-IG and numerous health insurance carriers (per their request) of all exclusion activity.

While strengthening our provider sanctions was a major step forward, we still needed additional ways to deal with the problems we faced. The Department addressed this need by also strengthening our provider enrollment provisions. Part 504 of our regulations defines a important concept - that is, the contractual nature of the relationship between providers and the Medicaid program. At one point, Medicaid was looked on as an entitlement program for providers in New York. That is no longer the case.

Enrollment applications require more information, get more extensive review and in many cases are denied when they are not in compliance with the requirements set forth in Part 504. The Department believes this has prevented many problematic providers the opportunity to defraud Medicaid. Part 504 also allows the Department the ability to terminate its contractual relationship with providers within 30 days upon written notice and without cause. However, in utilizing this provision, the Department has chosen to present providers with the reasons for its decision to terminate. An administrative hearing is not required. Providers terminated using this mechanism cannot be paid by Medicaid but are not subject to other restrictions. The employment of these regulations have been vigorously contested, but the Department has been extremely successful and landmark caselaw has been made in cases which reached the U.S. Court of Appeals.

In New York, providers do have the ability to voluntarily withdraw from Medicaid. This is not an administrative tool that we often utilize nor do we permit it in situations that we feel are particularly egregious. It is mostly likely to occur after a final determination to exclude the provider was already made and the Department and the provider have moved to the administrative hearing stage. If a problem arises with the presentation of the Department's case, it may be decided that accepting the provider's voluntary withdrawal may be the best resolution.

In conclusion, I would like to say that in New York we have implemented regulations that allow us to "stop the bleeding" while still recognizing providers rights to due process. However, we believe that administrators must build the regulatory capability to quickly move against problem providers. It is also important that state Medicaid agencies, Mediaid Fraud Control Units and HHS-IG have on-line access to a national database of provider activity.

Mr. Chairman, this concludes my remarks. I will be pleased to answer any questions.

Background

In State Fiscal Year 1994-95 New York expended approximately $20 billion (in federal, state and local funds) for the medical assistance (Medicaid) program to cover approximately 1.9 million recipients. Estimates of the amount of fraud, abuse and waste in the program run as high as 10% and the administration has made fighting fraud and protecting program integrity a top priority. In New York this is the responsibility of many agencies which include the Office of Inspector General for HHS, the various offices of the U.S. Attorney, the FBI, and the State Attorney General (Medicaid Fraud Control Unit). As the single state agency responsible for the administration of the Medicaid program, the New York State Department of Social Services has played the major role in combating fraud and in achieving savings through improvements in program integrity. The Department is staffed with auditors, investigators and medical professionals to carry out its functions.

Unfortunately, in New York, what we have seen especially in low income, economically depressed areas is that the business of Medicaid is flourishing. This activity replaces the intended provision of quality, accessible care. At the heart of this business is an entrepreneur, who may or not be a medical professional, and someone (a physician or a registered physician's assistant) who would see patients and/or order medically unnecessary tests, services and medications.

Medicaid has been billed fraudulently or unnecessarily through a variety of schemes used by labs, entrepreneurs, pharmacies and others. The labs bought blood from drug addicts, purchased or otherwise obtained legitimate Medicaid provider and client billing information from sources in the provider community, and simply "created" a paper trail of high cost lab orders and test results to support their billings. Often laboratories worked with unscrupulous clinic owners (entrepreneurs) who were more than willing to feed the labs the blood they desperately needed and to direct the physicians they hired to "pad" their orders for lab services, presumably in return for free help, office space or kickbacks. Some of the labs even went so far as to redesign their order forms so that expensive and unusual tests were batched or grouped with routine inexpensive tests. In that way, a mere one or two check marks in boxes on order forms created hundreds of dollars worth of unnecessary lab services.

In order to lend some degree of legitimacy to what they were doing and to generate more billings, the entrepreneurs needed physicians to order the services and write prescriptions. For the most part, the physicians hired were outside the regular medical establishment neither having hospital admitting privileges nor belonging to medical societies. Working in these pill-mills afforded these doctors a steady, heavy volume of patients for which they could bill Medicaid.

However, in some cases, the physicians had legitimate, thriving practices in other parts of the city and in the suburbs. All that was required was that they spend a minimal amount of time at a facility seeing "patients". The operators later found their purposes were better served hiring registered physician's assistants (RPAs) who were supposedly supervised by a physician. For the facilities which used the RPAs, the physician only had to come once a week and sign blank lab and prescription forms which would later be completed by clinic personnel. The scenario was such that a pharmacist or lab could bill Medicaid because they "only followed what the doctor had written or ordered". Clinic managers would point to the physician and claim that the individual who was treating the patients was the best or the only judge of what was medically necessary or appropriate.

When confronted, physicians would protest that the treatment they had given was appropriate and that they were unaware of any questionable practices at the facility. Yet they worked at clinics which were filthy, often without even sinks or toilets. Some locations had broken waste pipes running through so-called examining rooms. Most facilities lacked even the bare essentials of a legitimate medical practice, including an examining table and basic equipment. These physicians not only were unaffected by the conditions, they also failed to realize (if you were to believe them) that every person they saw day after day had the same complaints, asked for the same medications, and were required to submit to the same battery of tests. They never questioned why patients were not allowed to see them until they gave blood. They claimed that all they were attempting to do was provide much needed medical care to the poor and helpless, and were unaware of and uninvolved in any other matters at the clinic.

Substance abusers shopped for physicians and clinics willing to provide them with prescriptions for items that had a street value. Word quickly spread on the streets as to which doctors and/or clinics would provide such prescriptions, and also which pharmacies would fill them without asking any questions. Many clinics were in fact working directly with specific pharmacies and patients would be directed to go to that specific store. Pharmacies (some directly controlled by the entrepreneurs) seized the opportunity to make money in several ways. First of all, they would simply accept and fill the prescriptions as written. Earning the reputation on the street as a willing participant meant heavy volume and a profitable Medicaid business. With the tremendous increase in the number of individuals involved in the scam called "playing-the-doctor", a black market for drug wholesalers quickly became a major enterprise. Networks were set up between labs, pill-mills, and pharmacies. Individuals known as "non-men" (as in non-controlled substances) appeared on the streets purchasing the drugs that the individual had just obtained from a pharmacy. The substance abuser used the cash to buy illicit drugs and the cycle was repeated.

Today, the "non-men" are part of a larger network. The diverted drugs are collected, often packaged in baggies and re-sold at prices much lower than wholesale. Thus, an illegal wholesale and distribution business exists where drugs find their way back into small independent pharmacies only to be dispensed and then billed to Medicaid over and over again. A growing problem is that these diverted drugs often are being shipped out of the United State to a foreign country. From our perspective, this is the fastest growing Medicaid problem in New York and as a result, we are currently working with the FBI, other federal agencies and other State agencies to specifically address this problem. Hopefully, the end result will be to once and for all identify and put out of business the major rings that operate and control these diverted drugs and to exclude from the health care programs those who illegally buy these drugs off the street and resell them.

While historically the Department took steps to exclude or disqualify egregious providers participating in the types of schemes described above from Medicaid, we found that loopholes existed which allowed these same individuals to continue to harm the program. For example, excluded physicians would be unable to submit bills to Medicaid for services rendered but were easily able to continue writing orders for medically unnecessary items. Pharmacies, labs, and durable medical equipment dealers would fill the ders and claim entitlement to reimbursement because they had had no way of knowing the order writer had been excluded.

In New York, the administrative sanctioning process has been evolutionary, responding to the need to plug loopholes such as the one described above and restrict the ability of individuals to carry out their schemes to take advantage of the program. Administrators have worked to develop a process which allows the Department to react quickly to "stop the bleeding" while at the same time affording due process to providers.

New York Administrative Remedies

The Administration recognized the need for an aggressive up-front approach to effectively address the issue of Medicaid fraud and abuse. The resources and tools utilized by the Department include the exclusion of providers from Medicaid, enforcing the contractual nature of the relationship between providers and the Department, tightening the enrollment process and working closer with other oversight agencies.

The primary sanctioning authority for the Department is Part 515 of the Social Services regulations. N.Y. Comp. Codes R.&Regs. tit.18, Sec. 515.1 et seq. (1988). Part 515 defines the Department's authority, sets forth the requirements and procedures for sanctioning persons, recovering overpayments resulting from unacceptable practices, obtaining restitution, administrative appeals of sanctions and overpayments and reinstatement to the Medicaid program. Unacceptable practices are defined under 515.2 and include the following:

- false claims

- false statements

- failure to disclose

- converting a medical assistance payment to a use other than the use intended by the medical assistance program

- bribes and kickbacks

- unacceptable recordkeeping

- employment of sanctioned persons

- receiving additional payments, gifts, donations in addition to the amount paid under the program for any medical care, services or supplies.

- client deception

- excessive services

- failure to meet recognized standards

- unlawful documentation

- factoring

- solicitation of clients

- verification of MA eligibility and

- denial of services

This listing has evolved to meet the regulatory needs of the Department in order to address aberrant provider behavior. Beyond exclusion, Section 515.3 also authorizes the Department to impose limited participation. For example, this authority has been used to require pre-audits of claims or restrict physicians to practicing only at certain facilities and not allow them independent practice. This section also allows the Department to sanction an individual affiliated with a person or provider who has been already sanctioned themselves when the questioned conduct was accomplished within the course of duties of the person to be sanctioned and the other person knew of, should have known of, or consented to the conduct. New York has used this provision in regards to owners of businesses, lab medical directors and supervising pharmacists among others.

In New York the review of provider activity basically follows an audit protocol. In most cases, we will conduct entrance and exit conferences with the provider and employ sampling methodologies. An audit report will be prepared and forwarded to the provider detailing our initial findings, and the ramifications of those findings (i.e., the dollar value of any potential overpayment and/or the administrative sanction that the

Department intends to impose). The provider has thirty (30) days to respond to these findings. After analyzing the response a final report will be forwarded to the provider informing them of our determination. This report also serves as official notice of:
any administration actions,

- when the sanction will be effective (normally twenty (20) days from the date of notice),

- that their name will appear on a monthly list of providers not permitted to order or prescribe services or supplies reimbursed by Medicaid, and

- the providers right to challenge the action by requesting an administrative hearing within sixty (60) days of the notice.

In order to attack the problem of medically unnecessary orders for supplies and services, the Department utilizes a staff of medical professionals. When we have targeted a Medicaid-mill type physician or one whose volume of orders seems to be out of line with his/her peer group, we normally will have a nurse review 25 medical charts. The findings of this review will be sent to the physician in the same manner as the audit report. In this process, however, the Department forwards the physician's response along with our findings to a physician peer reviewer for final adjudication. If the peer reviewer feels the Department's initial findings are correct and if the citations are deemed serious enough, a final notice with sanction that mirrors the final audit report discussed previously, will be sent.

During the past five years, the Department has taken the following number of actions to exclude providers:

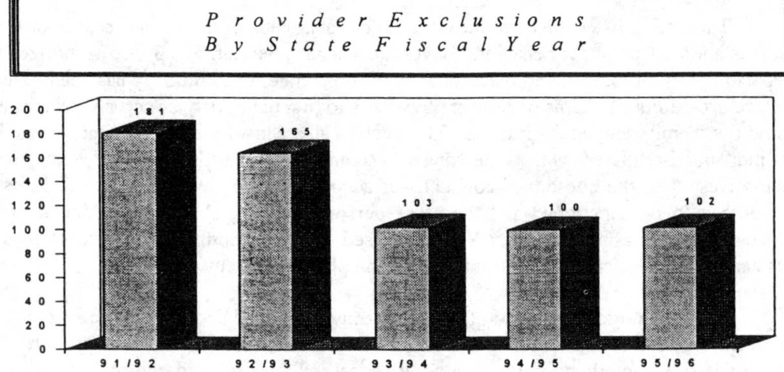

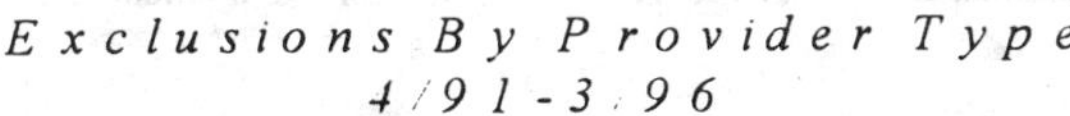

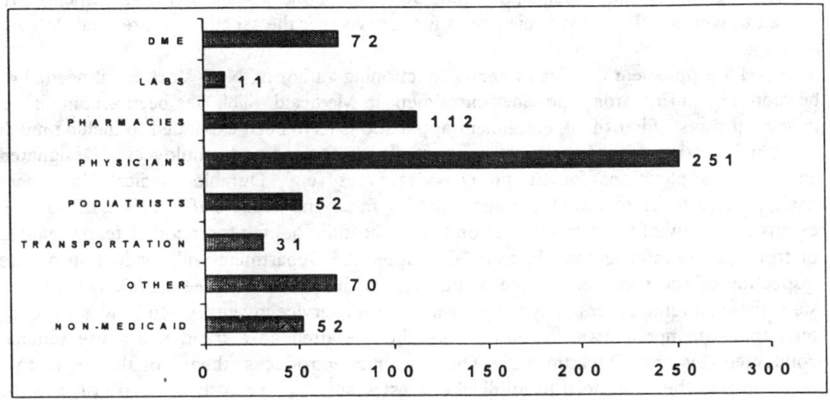

As mentioned previously, the provider is notified that their name will appear on a monthly listing (known as the PVR 292). This list is distributed to all providers who fill orders for supplies and services. In addition, the Department provides access to this information through an Electronic Medicaid Eligibility System (EMEVS). The intent is to put the Medicaid provider community on notice that the providers shown have been sanctioned by the Department and that any affiliation which affects Medicaid payments will be at the provider's risk (the least of which would be non-payment of claims). The basis for this action is in Section 515.5 of our regulations which prohibit payment to or on behalf of a person for any medical care, services or supplies furnished or ordered/prescribed by that person or under the supervision of that person during the period of exclusion.

In the course of conducting our business we often encounter scenarios where the ability to take an immediate action to sanction a provider is necessary. There are two major categories of activity where this would apply. The first is when the Department makes a determination that the public health or welfare, or that of a recipient, would be imminently endangered by the continued participation of the person/provider in the program. We often encounter this situation in the course of doing our medical reviews or during our undercover investigative activities. Referrals are made to any appropriate governmental oversight agency for their action as well. In these cases, the exclusion is effective until the conditions that caused the exclusion are corrected.

The second category has to do with situations where providers have been indicted or convicted of crimes relating to the provision of or participation in the performance of management or administrative services related to furnishing medical care, supplies or services.

Providers who have received an immediate sanction have the right to submit written arguments and documents within 30 days of the action. Their arguments are limited to whether there was a mistake of fact or whether the sanction was reasonable.

To supplement the Department's sanctioning authority, New York felt it needed to be more vigilant regarding provider enrollment in Medicaid. This has been accomplished in several ways. First of all, enrollment applications have been expanded to include much more information regarding the business itself, affiliations and employees. Designated enrollment applications for certain provider types (e.g., Durable Medical Equipment dealers) have to be reviewed and approved by fraud and abuse staff. This staff does an extensive review of the data supplied on the application looking for incomplete, misleading or troublesome information. In many situations, the Department will conduct an on-site inspection of the provider's office or business to insure that it meets basic Department standards including accessibility for patients and full-service inventory. In New York City, physicians are not allowed to enroll until they've attended a fraud and abuse seminar conducted by the Department. This seminar introduces them to the regulatory requirements they will need to fulfill, the latest scams they need to be aware of, and the ramifications of being sanctioned by the Department.

Enrollment applications may be denied by the Department under Part 504 of our regulations which establishes the contractual nature of the relationship between providers and the Department. Denials may be for a number of reasons including: false representation or omission of material facts, previous or current exclusion from Medicaid in any state of the United States, not having made restitution for prior Medicaid overpayments, a prior finding of engaging in an unacceptable practice in Medicaid or Medicare, failure to supply requested information or lack of proper licensing or certification. Providers are given written notification of the denial stating the reasons. The applicant has the right to appeal the denial by filing a reconsideration request within 45 days of the notice. The Department will review any documents submitted in support of the application and issue a written determination after reconsideration within 30 days of the receipt of the request. The chart below highlights the number of denials the Department has issued during the past five years.

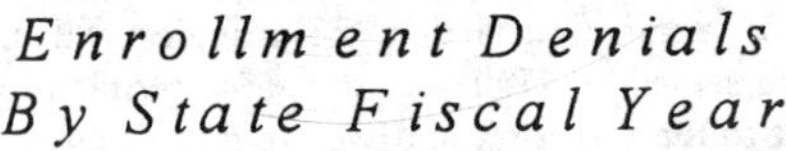

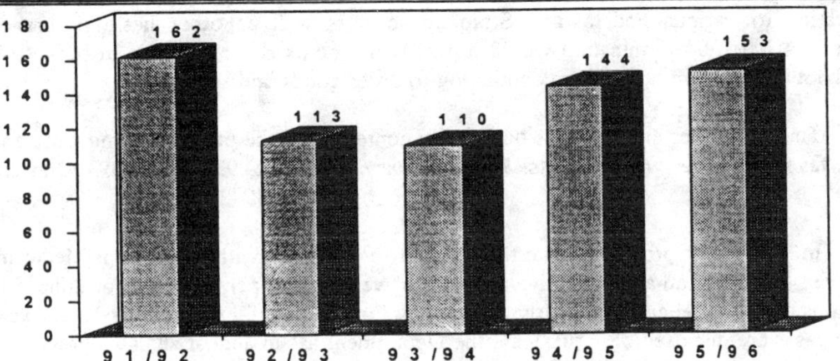

This intensive enrollment review process has been highly effective in allowing the Department to gather and analyze as much information as possible prior to accepting a provider's application to participate in Medicaid. With our experience and our data bases we have been able to profile troublesome situations and believe we have denied many individuals the opportunity to defraud the Medicaid program.

The Department's ability to do this has not been implemented without contention. In fact, it has been vigorously contested in both state and federal courts. We have been extremely successful in these forums and landmark caselaw has been made in many cases which reached either the U.S. Court of Appeals or the State Court of Appeals. For example in Senape v. Constantino, 936 F.2d 687 (2nd cir. 1991), the Department successfully defended its right to utilize its enrollment process to ensure that problematic providers are not granted a contract to participate in Medicaid.

It has been our experience that emphasizing the contractual nature of the relationship between providers and the Department, developing regulations which clearly define the nature and expectations of this contractual relationship, as well as to whom it applies, and aggressively enforcing these provisions has been a very successful approach to dealing with troublesome providers. New York has utilized these regulations to deal with aberrant providers in a much less time consuming way than the traditional audit/exclusion process.

In situations where we see aberrant practices but have not detected fraud (which would result in a referral to the Medicaid Fraud Control Unit within the Attorney General's Office), these provisions may be applied. The approach is basic, the Department decides to terminate its contractual relationship with the provider. This termination can be effective upon 30 days written notice and without cause. However, as a matter of policy the Department has chosen it submit to providers the basis for its decision to terminate. The effect of this type of termination is that the provider will no longer be eligible to receive Medicaid reimbursement. Utilizing this 504 termination means we are <u>not</u> charging an overpayment to the provider, and we are not officially excluding the provider from participating in Medicaid with all the ramifications that go with that, such as notification to various Federal and State agencies as well as other health insurance carriers. A Part 504 termination would normally not be used for a physician because it would not prevent him or her from continuing to order goods and services.

This is another area that has been hotly contested by the provider community and where favorable caselaw now exists, 701 Pharmacy v. Perales, 933 F.2d 1093 (2nd cir. 1991).

In New York providers have the ability to voluntarily withdrawn from Medicaid. However, this is not an administrative action that we normally permit. It is not utilized in situations that we feel are particularly egregious. For the handful of providers every year whose cases are disposed of in this way, the Department has in almost all cases previously issued an exclusion and notified HHS. We may at some later point (prior to or during the administrative hearing) because aware of a problem with the presentation of our case.

Notification

The Department routinely notifies the New York Regional Office for the Department of Health and Human Services (HHS) Office of Inspector General for all exclusions. What we submit is in fact a copy of the notice that we send to the Medicaid provider. New York routinely receives notice from HHC of exclusion actions taken by the Federal agency. New York will post that information to our provider file database. Providers are then sent a notice from the Department notifying that they are being excluded from participating in Medicaid in New York as a result of the Federal action and for a period to coincide with the Federal period of exclusion. A copy of this provider notification is also sent to HHS-OIG regional office in New York to notify them that the Department has followed up on the Federal action.

Recommendations

While the administrative process varies state to state, we believe the following recommendations have value for both federal and state agencies:

- There is a need for a national data bank of exclusion activity. State Medicaid agencies, Medicaid Fraud Control Units, HCFA and HHS-IG should all have on-line access to conviction and exclusion information.

- Federal and State agencies should take the necessary steps to define the contractual terms of their relationship with Medicaid providers utilizing the caselaw that already has been established.

- Health care providers who are permitted to write prescriptions or order goods and services need to be held accountable for the medical necessity of those items regardless of whether or not they themselves received reimbursement.

Conclusion

We believe that in order to fight Medicaid fraud and protect program integrity, agencies at the state and federal level must have regulatory capability and flexibility to enable the administrative sanctioning of providers to be an effective process. We also believe that to be truly effective the sanctioning process must be supplemented with the ability to prevent problematic providers from enrolling in the first instance and also with ability of oversight agencies to quickly terminate their relationship with providers. In New York we have implemented regulations that allow us to "stop the bleeding" while still recognizing and addressing providers rights to due process.

Mr. SHAYS. Thank you, Mr. White. Dr. Koontz.

Dr. KOONTZ. Mr. Chairman, members of the subcommittee, ladies and gentlemen, I'm Dr. Warren Koontz, executive director of the Virginia Board of Medicine.

On behalf of the Department of Health Professions and the Board of Medicine of the Commonwealth of Virginia, I want to thank you for inviting me to participate in this discussion on the processes followed by Federal and State agencies to exclude fraudulent providers from Medicaid and other Federal health care programs.

The Virginia Board of Medicine is 1 of 12 boards within the Department of Health Professions, an agency under the Secretary of Health and Human Resources for the Commonwealth.

The Board of Medicine regulates over 26,000 practitioners licensed or certified in Virginia. These practitioners not only include doctors of medicine and osteopathy but also doctors of podiatry and chiropractic. In addition, we regulate physical therapists, physician assistants, acupuncturists, respiratory therapists, occupational therapists, rad techs, and licensed acupuncturists.

The Virginia Department of Health Professions and the Board of Medicine work in concert to provide an optimal regulatory system to promote the safe and effective delivery of health care to the citizens of the Commonwealth by licensing applicants who meet minimum qualifications as determined by law and regulations.

Taking appropriate action to enforce compliance with legal requirements, issuing licenses or permits to certain health care regulated businesses and inspecting for compliance with laws and regulations, studying and recommending the appropriate degree of regulation of health professions and occupations.

Our duties are to review the qualifications and issue licenses or certificates to qualified health care professionals; to provide accurate, timely resolution of complaints; to provide timely, cost-effective access to accurate information concerning licensure, disciplinary actions and the regulatory system.

To adjudicate violations of statutes and regulations and to anticipate the dynamic environment of the health care industry and develop appropriate legislation and regulatory initiatives.

The Board of Medicine has 17 members appointed by the Governor, including 11 doctors of medicine, an osteopath, a chiropractor, a podiatrist, a clinical psychologist and two public members.

The vast majority of complaints that come to the Board of Medicine are written, but a few do come by newspaper articles or telephone.

The source of these complaints are many; the largest majority being from consumers, but a number, however, come from other governmental agencies, both Federal and State, the Department of Health and law enforcement, to give an example.

In a 5-year period, the Board of Medicine received and investigated over 4,000 complaints, the largest number of these with the primary complaint being standard of care, over 2,000. Almost 1,000 were unprofessional conduct, and by fraud as being the primary or the first cause of the complaint was only 104.

When a complaint is lodged against a practitioner regulated by the Board of Medicine, an investigation is conducted by the enforcement division of the Department of Health Professions. Depending on the nature of the allegations, these investigations may be conducted cooperatively with the Virginia State Police, the Drug Enforcement Agency or the Medicaid Fraud Control Unit.

An investigative report is developed and, after completion, it is submitted to the board for its review. If an apparent violation of law or regulation is identified, the case is, under the Virginia Administrative Process Act, referred for an informal conference.

The informal conference committee is made up of three members of the Board of Medicine who review the investigative report and discuss the facts with the respondent, who may or may not have an attorney.

The informal conference committee, by law, has the ability to dismiss the allegations, issue a reprimand or place the practitioner on probation.

If the allegations are substantial and is thought by the three-member committee that a suspension or a revocation of the license may be in order, the allegations are referred to the board for approval for the holding of a formal administrative hearing.

A formal hearing panel is made up of at least five members of the Board of Medicine, and this panel has the authority to dismiss the allegations, issue a reprimand, put the license on probation, or to suspend or revoke the license.

The Virginia statutes also provide authority to the board to take disciplinary action without a hearing in several instances.

The Board of Medicine, under Virginia Code, has the ability to summarily suspend the license of a practitioner if there is evidence that there is a substantial danger to the public, health, or safety which warrants this action.

In addition, the code also allows for suspension or revocation of a license upon notification that a person licensed to practice any of the healing arts in the Commonwealth has had his license to practice that branch of the healing arts revoked or suspended in another State or territories.

Similar mandatory action is authorized for licensees who have been convicted of a felony or those who have been adjudged legally incompetent.

In fact, those practitioners who engage in fraudulent conduct can be found guilty of a number of violations of the Virginia Code. I won't go through those. They are in your statement.

Following the entry of an order which encumbers a license, whether it be reprimand, probation, revocation, or suspension, the final order is public information and is sent to those parties specifically requesting such information and to a standard mailing list which includes the National Practitioner Data Bank, Federation of State Medical Boards for doctors of medicine and osteopathy and other federations such as the podiatric, osteopathic, chiropractic, et cetera.

At the present time, the Board of Medicine does share information on disciplinary action, in addition to the previously named entities, also with liability insurance carriers, health insurance carriers, other licensed jurisdictions, the hospitals in Virginia, the

State Hospital Association, Department of Health and Human Services, Medicare and Medicaid Intermediaries and the Drug Enforcement Agency.

On a weekly basis, the board provides notices of administrative proceedings and orders to our State Physicians Review Organization.

The committee may wish to contact the Federation of State Medical Boards of the United States. The federation could provide you more information on its new computer system, which is to become operational and give on-line access for all 68 boards of medicine and osteopathy in the section several months.

The Virginia Board of Medicine believes that its relationships with Federal agencies and other State agencies are good. The Department of Health Professions is beginning its implementation stage of a re-engineering process that has been going on for the past 9 months.

At the conclusion of this last phase, there should be an increased ability to transmit and share data, adjudicate cases, and provide faster communication with local, State, and Federal agencies.

The Board of Medicine appreciates the opportunity to speak with you today and would be happy to work with this committee to help in any way that you feel is appropriate. And I thank you.

[The prepared statement of Dr. Koontz follows:]

Thursday, September 5, 1996

Chairman Christopher Shays

Members of the Subcommittee on Human Resources and Intergovernmental Relations

Ladies and Gentlemen:

I am Dr. Warren Koontz, MD, Executive Director of the Virginia Board of
Medicine. On behalf of the Department of Health Professions and the Board of
Medicine of the Commonwealth of Virginia, I want to thank you for inviting me to
participate in this discussion on the processes followed by federal and state agencies to
exclude fraudulent providers from Medicaid and other federal health care programs.
The Virginia Board of Medicine is one of 12 boards within the Department of Health
Professions, an agency under the Secretary of Health and Human Resources for the
Commonwealth of Virginia. The Board of Medicine regulates the practice of over
26,000 practitioners licensed or certified in Virginia. These practitioners include not
only doctors of medicine and osteopathy, but also doctors of podiatry and chiropractic.
In addition, the Board of Medicine regulates physical therapists, physician assistants,
acupuncturists, respiratory therapists, occupational therapists, radiological technology
practitioners, and licensed acupuncturists.

The Virginia Department of Health Professions and the Board of Medicine work
in concert to provide an optimal regulatory system.

The mission of the Virginia Department of Health Professions is to promote the
safe and effective delivery of health care to the citizens of the Commonwealth by
(1) licensing applicants who meet minimum qualifications as determined by law and

regulation, (2) taking appropriate action to enforce compliance with legal requirements, (3) issuing licenses or permits to certain health regulated businesses and inspecting for compliance with applicable laws and regulations, and (4) studying and recommending the appropriate degree of regulation of health professions and occupations. The Board of Medicine's duties are: (1) to review qualifications and issue licenses or certificates to qualified health care professionals; (2) to provide appropriate, timely resolution of complaints; (3) to provide timely, cost effective access to accurate information concerning licensure, disciplinary actions, and the regulatory system; (4) to adjudicate violations of statutes and regulations; (5) to anticipate the dynamic environment of the health care industry and develop appropriate legislation and regulatory initiatives. The Board of Medicine has 17 members including 11 doctors of medicine, one osteopath, one chiropractor, one podiatrist, a clinical psychologist, and two public members.

The vast majority of complaints to the Board of Medicine are written, but a few come by telephone or newspaper articles. The source of these complaints are numerous; the largest majority being from consumers. A number, however, are from other governmental agencies, both federal and state, the Department of Health, and law enforcement. To give an example:

1991-1996

Complaints Received by the Board of Medicine	4,017
Standard of Care Complaints	2,260
Unprofessional Conduct	877
Fraud	104

When a complaint is lodged against a practitioner regulated by the Board of Medicine, an investigation is conducted by the Enforcement Division of the Department of Health Professions. Depending on the nature of the allegations, these investigations may be conducted cooperatively with the Virginia State Police, the DEA or the Medicaid Fraud Control Unit. An investigative report is developed and, after completion, is submitted to the Board of Medicine for its review. If an apparent violation of law or regulation is identified, the case is, under the Virginia Administrative Process Act, referred for an informal conference. The informal conference committee is made up of three members of the Board of Medicine who review the investigative report and discuss the facts with the respondent who may have an attorney. The informal conference committee, by law, has the ability to dismiss the allegations, issue a reprimand, or to place the practitioner on probation. If the allegations are substantial and it is thought by the three-member committee that a suspension or revocation of the license may be in order, the allegations are referred to the Board for approval for the holding of a formal administrative hearing. A formal hearing panel is made up of at least five members of the Board of Medicine and this panel has the authority to dismiss the allegations, issue a reprimand, put the license on probation, or to suspend or revoke the license.

The Virginia statutes also provide authority for the Board to take disciplinary action without a hearing in several instances. The Board of Medicine, under Virginia Code §54.1-2920 has the ability to summarily suspend the license of a practitioner if there is evidence that there is a substantial danger to the public, health, or safety which warrants this action. In addition, Virginia Code §54.1-2917 requires mandatory suspension or revocation of a license upon notification that any person licensed to practice any of the healing arts in the Commonwealth has had his license to practice that branch of the healing arts revoked or suspended in another state, the District of Columbia, or a United States possession or territory, or a foreign jurisdiction. Similar mandatory action is authorized for licensees who have been convicted of a felony or those who have been adjudged legally incompetent. Virginia Code §54.1-2409 gives the Director of the Department of Health Professions the same authority to mandatorily suspend a license, and the Director takes this action when the Board is not in session.

The practitioner who engages in fraudulent conduct could be found guilty of the following violations of the Medical Practice Act, Virginia Code §54.1-2914, Unprofessional Conduct: (a) Section A.9., "conducts his practice in a manner contrary to the standards of ethics of his branch of the healing arts"; (b) Section A.13. "performs any act likely to deceive, defraud or harm the public"; (c) Section A.14. "violates any provision of statute or regulation, state or federal, relating to the manufacture, distribution, dispensing or administration of drugs"; (d) Section A.15. "violates or cooperates with others in violating any of the provisions of this chapter or regulations of the Board." Further, Virginia Code §54.1-2915 states that the Board may suspend for a stated period of time or indefinitely, or revoke any certificate or license or censure or reprimand any person or place him on probation for such time as it may designate for several causes; among them are:

- False statements or representations or fraud or deceit in obtaining admission to the practice, or fraud or deceit in the practice of any branch of the healing arts;

- Unprofessional conduct as defined in this chapter;

- Restriction of a license to practice a branch of the healing arts in another state, the District of Columbia, a United States possession or territory, or a foreign jurisdiction.

Virginia Code §54.1-2916, in relevant part, states that the Board may suspend or revoke any certificate or license if it finds that the candidate, applicant or licensee:

A.1.   Has been convicted in any state, territory or country of any felony or of any crime involving moral turpitude;

B.   The conviction of an offense in another state, territory or country, which if committed in Virginia would be a felony, shall be treated as a felony conviction under this section regardless of its designation in the other state, territory or country.

Following the entry of an Order which encumbers a license, whether it be a reprimand, probation, revocation or suspension, the final Order is public information and is sent to both parties specifically requesting such information and to a standard mailing list which includes the National Data Practitioner Bank and Federation of State Medical Boards (for the doctors of medicine and osteopathy). Other practitioners regulated by the Board of Medicine will have their orders forwarded to their appropriate federation, such as the Federation of Podiatric Boards, the Federation of Osteopathic Boards, Federation of Chiropractic Boards, or the Federation of Physical Therapist Association, etc. At the present time the Virginia Board of Medicine does share information on disciplinary action, in addition to the previously named entities, also with liability insurance carriers, health insurance carriers, other licensed jurisdictions, the hospitals in Virginia, the State Hospital Association, Department of Health and Human Services, Medicare and Medicaid Intermediaries, and the Drug Enforcement Agency. On a weekly basis, the Board provides notices of administrative proceedings and orders to the State PRO, Virginia Health Quality Center.

The committee may wish to contact the Federation of State Medical Boards of the United States, Inc. at Federation Place, 400 Fuller Wiser Road, Suite 300, Euless, TX 76039-3855, phone number (817) 868-4000 or fax (817) 868-4099. The Federation of State Medical Boards could provide complete information on its new computer system, which is to become operational and give online access for all 68 boards of medicine and osteopathy in the next several months.

The Virginia Board of Medicine believes that its relationships with federal agencies and other state agencies are good. The Department of Health Professions is beginning its implementation stage of a reengineering process that has been going on for the past nine months. At the conclusion of this last phase there should be a increased ability to transmit and share data, adjudicate cases, and provide faster communication with local, state, and federal agencies.

The Board of Medicine of the Commonwealth of Virginia appreciates the opportunity to speak with you today, and would be happy to work with this committee to help in any way that you feel is appropriate. Thank you.

MEDICAID EXCLUDED PROVIDER PROCESS

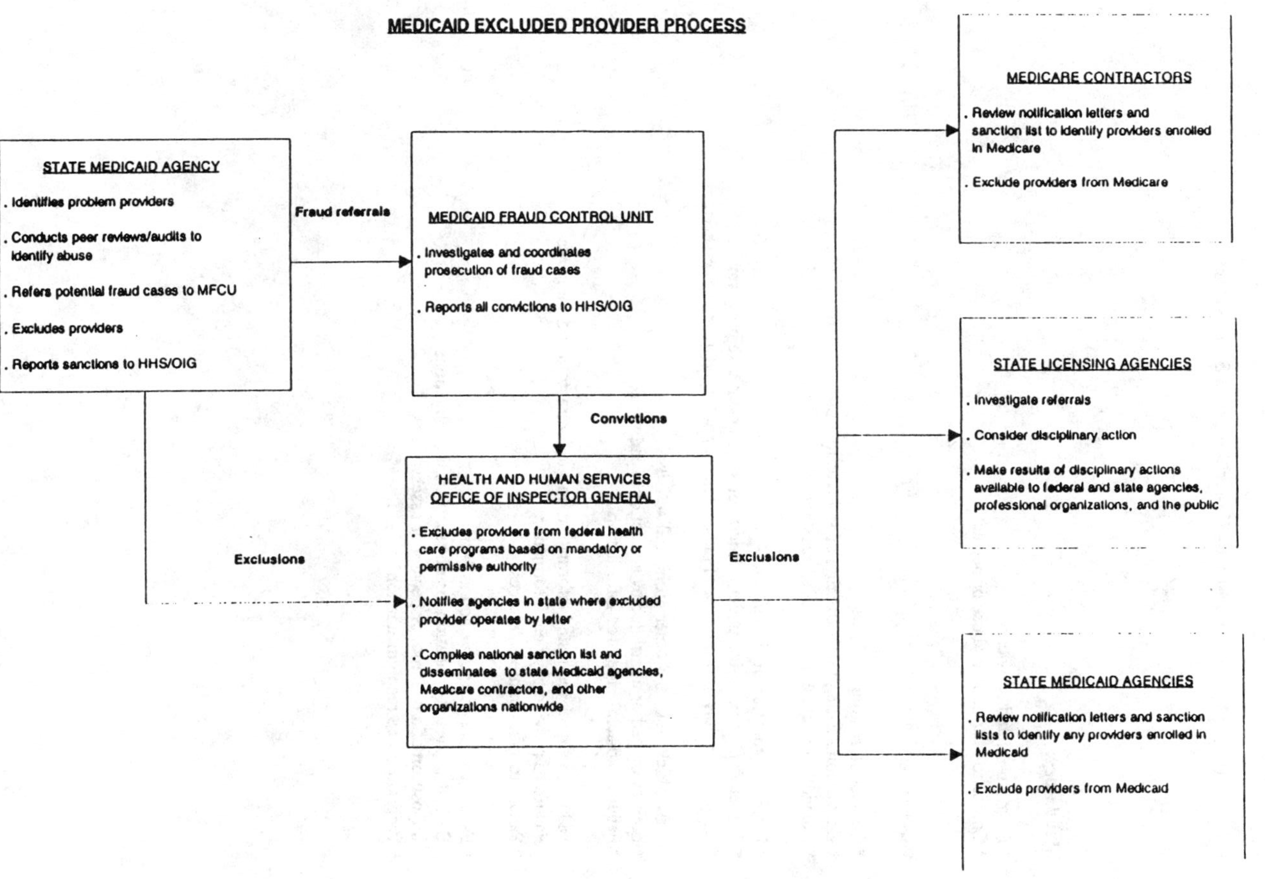

Exclusions Under the Social Security Act

Mandatory:

* Program-related conviction
* Conviction for patient abuse or neglect

Permissive:

* Conviction relating to fraud
* Conviction relating to obstruction of an investigation
* Conviction relating to controlled substances

* License revocation or suspension
* Suspension or exclusion under a federal or state health care program
* Excessive claims or furnishing of unnecessary or substandard items or services

* Fraud, kickbacks and other prohibited activity
* Entities owned or controlled by a sanctioned individual
* Failure to disclose required information

* Failure to supply requested information on subcontractors and suppliers
* Failure to provide payment information
* Failure to grant immediate access

* Failure to take corrective action
* Default on health education loan or scholarship obligations
* Imposition of a civil money penalty or assessment
* Program office recommendation

Mr. Chairman and Members of the Subcommittee:

I am pleased to be here today to discuss our ongoing work related to health care providers who have been removed from their state Medicaid programs for committing program fraud or rendering substandard care to beneficiaries. When this occurs, the Department of Health and Human Services' (HHS) Office of the Inspector General (OIG) is responsible for determining whether such circumstances warrant prompt nationwide exclusion of those providers from all federal health programs. Our work responds to your concern that despite the OIG's efforts, providers who have been convicted of fraud or who have delivered inadequate or inappropriate care may still be participating in these programs.

My comments today will focus on the process the OIG uses for excluding providers from Medicaid, Medicare, and other federal health programs. Our objective was to determine whether this process effectively ensures that excluded providers do not continue to participate in these programs.

In developing this information, we visited the District of Columbia, Illinois, Maryland, Missouri, and Virginia. For these five states,[1] we worked with officials of state Medicaid agencies, licensing boards, and Medicare contractors to document their exclusion processes. We performed computer matches of OIG and state lists of excluded providers and Medicare claims data. We also reviewed case files for a judgmentally selected sample of excluded providers to determine the nature of their wrongdoing and the types of sanctions they received. We also performed limited work in New York State to understand the state Medicaid program's exclusion process. In addition, we met with officials from the four OIG field offices--Chicago, New York, Philadelphia, and Washington, D.C.--that oversee these six states, and with OIG headquarters officials.

In brief, although the OIG has excluded thousands of providers, our work suggests that several weaknesses in its process can leave sanctioned providers on the rolls of federal health programs for unacceptable periods of time. This puts at risk the health and safety of beneficiaries and compromises the financial integrity of Medicaid, Medicare, and other federal health programs. The weaknesses we identified include (1) lengthy delays in the OIG's decision process, even in cases where a provider has been convicted of fraud or patient abuse or neglect; (2) inconsistencies among OIG field offices regarding which providers will be considered for nationwide exclusion; (3) states not informing the OIG about providers who agree to stop participating in their Medicaid programs even though the reason for agreeing to withdraw is sometimes egregious patient care or abusive billing; and (4) how

---

[1]For the purposes of this discussion, we include the District of Columbia as a state.

states use information from the OIG to remove excluded providers from state programs.

In addition to identifying these system weaknesses, we attempted to assess the magnitude of these problems. Incomplete records in the OIG field offices where we conducted work did not permit such an analysis, however. We therefore could not identify the universe of cases referred to the OIG field offices, determine if all cases received were reviewed and acted upon in a timely manner, or obtain the rationale for decisions not to recommend exclusion to headquarters.

BACKGROUND

Medicaid is a joint federal-state health program for the poor that expended $159 billion in fiscal year 1995 to provide health care coverage for over 40 million people. Because of its size and complex structure, Medicaid is vulnerable to fraud and abuse. State Medicaid agencies have the primary responsibility to protect the program's financial integrity and to ensure that beneficiaries have access to quality care. This includes ensuring that appropriate safeguards are in place to remove providers that commit fraud or abuse, or are incompetent, from state programs.

At the federal level, the Secretary of HHS has delegated to the OIG the authority under sections 1128 and 1156 of the Social Security Act to exclude health care providers from most federal health care programs.[2] The OIG, through its Office of Investigations, is required to exclude, nationwide, providers who have been convicted of Medicare- or Medicaid-related fraud and patient abuse or neglect, and felonies related to health care fraud and controlled substances.[3] These actions are termed "mandatory exclusions."

---

[2] OIG exclusions are effective with respect to Medicare (title XVIII of the Social Security Act) and state health care programs, defined as Medicaid (title XIX), Maternal and Child Health Services Block grant (title V), and Block Grants to States for Social Services (title XX). As a result of the Federal Acquisition Streamlining Act of 1994, which mandates and expands the governmentwide effect of all debarments, suspensions, and other exclusionary actions to federal procurement and nonprocurement programs, OIG exclusions also apply to health care providers participating in the Federal Employees' Health Benefits Program (FEHBP) administered by the U.S. Office of Personnel Management and the Civilian Health and Medical Program of the Uniformed Services (CHAMPUS) administered by the Department of Defense.

[3] These latter two mandatory exclusions were recently added by the Health Insurance Portability and Accountability Act of 1996.

The OIG also has authority to exclude other individuals or entities if the OIG determines that the particular facts in a case meet its criteria. These so-called "permissive exclusions" may be based on, for example, submitting excessive claims, license suspensions and revocations, and sanctions imposed by federal or state health agencies. (See the appendix for a complete list of exclusion authorities.)

The OIG field offices receive referrals of sanction actions taken by state Medicaid agencies, licensing boards, Medicaid fraud control units (MFCU),[4] and others. For mandatory cases, they assemble and forward to headquarters the case files containing evidence of a provider's criminal conviction. For referrals falling under the permissive exclusion authorities, the field offices receive documents related to disciplinary actions taken by state Medicaid agencies, licensing boards, or others. They assess the relevant facts and forward to OIG headquarters the cases they recommend for exclusion. OIG headquarters makes the final decision about whether to exclude the provider from program participation.

When the OIG excludes a provider, it sends notification letters to organizations such as state Medicaid agencies, Medicare claims-processing contractors, state licensing boards, and MFCUs in the states where the provider is known to practice or operate. When applicable, the provider's employer is also notified. In addition, information on excluded providers is disseminated nationally through monthly reports and semiannual cumulative listings.

As of February 1996--the latest date for which cumulative data were prepared--the OIG had excluded 8,830 providers from federal health care programs nationwide. Three exclusion categories-- conviction for program-related crime, conviction for patient abuse or neglect, and license suspensions and revocations--accounted for 76 percent of these nationwide exclusions.

OIG PROCESS DOES NOT ENSURE THAT ALL
PROVIDERS ARE EXCLUDED IN A TIMELY MANNER

In reviewing the OIG's exclusion of state-referred cases, we identified a number of cases--including those involving mandatory exclusions or serious quality of care issues--that remained unresolved for long periods of time. In the Chicago and Washington field offices, for example, we found delays that were due, at least in part, to state Medicaid agencies and MFCUs not always submitting

---

[4]Most states have MFCUs that must be organizationally independent of the agency that operates the state Medicaid program. A MFCU is usually a component of the state attorney general's office. MFCUs investigate and prosecute provider fraud and cases relating to neglect or abuse of patients in nursing homes and other facilities.

documentation the field offices needed to process the exclusion.
Thus, the completeness of the documentation provided by these
agencies varied, necessitating frequent back-and-forth telephone
contacts and correspondence to obtain data. The Washington field
office advised us that it could take as long as 2 months to obtain
needed documentation from state agencies.

In other instances, however, case files showed long periods of
inactivity with no apparent explanation for the delays. In one
case, a pharmacy was terminated for overbilling the Illinois
Medicaid program by over $117,000. It took the Chicago field
office 15 months to forward the case to headquarters for exclusion.
The case file showed no activity for extended periods of time,
including a 10-month period. In another case, the field office
referred a provider to headquarters for exclusion 19 months after
the Illinois MFCU notified it that the provider had pled guilty in
state court to falsely billing for Medicaid services. Two and one-
half months after the case was forwarded to OIG headquarters, the
provider was excluded nationwide.

INCONSISTENCIES AMONG FIELD OFFICES

Another weakness we identified in the OIG's process involves
inconsistencies among its field offices in how they use their
discretionary authority and the types of cases they refer to
headquarters. This is especially true in the case of permissive
exclusions, where the field offices may decide whether to recommend
exclusion.

In 1987, the OIG was given expanded discretionary authority to
exclude providers nationwide.[5] Our work to date, however,
indicates that the OIG has not always used its expanded exclusion
authority as widely as it could. OIG officials told us that given
the OIG's competing priorities, permissive exclusions have
sometimes taken a lower priority. In October 1992, the OIG
instructed its field offices to only process state Medicaid agency
and licensing board disciplinary actions in which there was actual
harm to patients and in which the provider had moved to another
state. Field offices asked state agencies to only report these
types of cases. About 1 year later, however, the OIG rescinded
this guidance and state agencies were asked to once again refer all
cases.

We also observed apparent inconsistencies in the way field
offices are processing permissive cases. As a result, providers
with equally serious problems could be treated differently by the
OIG depending on their location. For example, an official in the
Washington field office told us that the office would not consider

---

[5]Medicare and Medicaid Patient and Program Protection Act of 1987
(P.L. 100-93).

4

recommending nationwide exclusion unless the state Medicaid agency had excluded the provider, or a licensing board had revoked a license, for at least 1 year. The Chicago and New York field offices, however, use a 2-year rule of thumb.

<u>OIG NOT NOTIFIED OF CERTAIN WITHDRAWALS</u>
<u>FROM STATE MEDICAID PROGRAMS</u>

During our state visits we found that states were not always notifying the OIG of certain providers effectively excluded from the respective state's Medicaid program. One state we visited sometimes permits providers who are being considered for removal from their Medicaid programs to "voluntarily" withdraw rather than face formal sanction. Another state sometimes terminates on short notice providers it suspects of engaging in improper or inappropriate activities. Neither type of withdrawal is reported to the OIG. While this results in safeguards for those states' Medicaid programs and beneficiaries, it affords no protection for Medicare or other states' Medicaid programs.[6]

Illinois sometimes negotiates a settlement agreement with a provider against whom it has initiated termination proceedings. This effectively excludes the provider without the state having to spend the time and resources needed to pursue a formal action. In such an agreement, the provider admits to no wrongdoing but agrees to withdraw from participating in Medicaid. The provider also forfeits the right to appeal if denied reinstatement at a later date. The provider does not, however, face the prospect of losing his or her license to practice because, according to state Medicaid officials, the case is not referred to the state licensing board. In addition, the state does not report such a case to the OIG. This withdrawal process enables Illinois to remove providers from its Medicaid program relatively quickly and keep them out. But, because the state does not report these actions to the state licensing board or the OIG, the providers may continue to provide harmful, unnecessary, or excessive services to beneficiaries in other federal or state programs.

---

[6]Section 1902 of the Social Security Act requires the state Medicaid agency to report to HHS whenever a provider of services is terminated, suspended, or otherwise sanctioned or prohibited from participating in the program. HHS regulations define the term "otherwise sanctioned" as intending to cover all actions that limit the ability of a person to participate in the program regardless of what such an action is called, including situations in which an individual or entity voluntarily withdraws from a program to avoid a formal sanction (42 C.F.R. 1001.601). Furthermore, the provision regarding exclusion for loss of license also defines surrender of license to avoid an adverse action as grounds for exclusion.

Currently, about 23 percent of the physicians not allowed to participate in the Illinois Medicaid program have withdrawn in lieu of an action against them. We found that some of the providers who had withdrawn for what appeared to be serious quality of care problems were still able to bill Medicare in Illinois. For example, Medicare paid a podiatrist over $20,000 for services provided to program beneficiaries since he withdrew from the Illinois Medicaid program in August 1995. The podiatrist withdrew from the program after the state alleged that he had provided grossly inferior care to Medicaid recipients.

An Illinois Medicaid official told us that he did not believe that the settlement agreements preclude the state from formally referring withdrawals to outside organizations. If the state agency started to do so, however, he believed that providers would soon opt to pursue the formal sanction route rather than withdrawing. Consequently, the state might lose a valuable tool for removing undesirable providers from Medicaid and would be forced to spend more time pursuing exclusion. This official speculated that had Illinois not aggressively moved to remove these providers from the Medicaid program through voluntary withdrawals, the providers would still be in the program.

We do not know how prevalent voluntary withdrawals are nationwide. Most of the other states we visited told us they do not allow providers to withdraw from their programs to avoid formal sanction. Although New York sometimes allows providers to withdraw from its program, state Medicaid officials told us these cases are reported to the OIG, the state licensing board, and others. Certain providers New York suspects of abuse, however, are terminated but not reported to the OIG.

We were informed by New York officials that state program regulations permit either the provider or state Medicaid agency to terminate a provider's participation in the program upon 30 days' written notice. According to state officials, this practice has been used primarily against pharmacies that the state suspected were heavily involved in dispensing drugs with a street market. As a result, the state agency has been able to deal quickly with pharmacies that it believed were involved in drug diversion. Like voluntary withdrawals in Illinois, however, these cases are not reported to the OIG.

<u>STATES' USE OF THE OIG'S</u>
<u>EXCLUDED PROVIDER LISTS</u>

The OIG widely disseminates information on excluded providers through monthly reports and periodic cumulative listings to various state and federal agencies so that they, too, will remove these providers from their programs. We found, however, that for several reasons states sometimes have difficulty identifying and excluding providers who appear on the lists.

First, the states have difficulty identifying individuals--
such as nurses, pharmacists, or physicians--who are employed by
hospitals, nursing homes, pharmacies, and health maintenance
organizations that bill the program under the entities' billing
number. These providers, once sanctioned, can change employers or
move to other states and potentially continue to provide services
through federal health care programs without detection.

Second, providers sometimes are not identified because states
tend to use the OIG's monthly list for a onetime check against
their active provider files. However, they may not review prior
monthly lists to check a provider who applies for program
participation in a subsequent month. Thus, a provider could later
enroll in the state's Medicaid program after being excluded
nationwide by the OIG and not be detected.

Finally, some states do not always check providers appearing
on the list who have out-of-state addresses. An official in
Missouri, for example, told us that although they check the OIG
monthly list with in-state and border state addresses, they do not
check names from other states. New York officials also told us
that it would be time-consuming to check the list of their Medicaid
providers against the entire OIG list each month; instead, they
only check for New York addresses. In addition, they said the
OIG's cumulative list is cumbersome to use and the information is
not formatted in a way that would permit a large state, such as New
York, to match provider names.

When we performed a computer match of the OIG exclusion list
to Illinois' enrolled provider file, we found 13 out-of-state
providers who had been excluded by the OIG between 1988 and 1995
but who were still enrolled in the Illinois Medicaid program. One
of them had received almost $25,000 in Medicaid payments since
being excluded by the OIG. Although the others had not billed the
program since they were excluded by the OIG, state Medicaid
officials acknowledged that they would have been paid had they
submitted claims.

<u>MAGNITUDE OF PROBLEM</u>
<u>COULD NOT BE DETERMINED</u>

Although we attempted to identify the magnitude and
pervasiveness of problems in the exclusion process, we were unable
to do so--primarily because of a lack of case file documentation at
the OIG field offices.

In our visits to OIG field offices, we found that they were
not always able to fully account for the number of referrals they
received from the states. For example, the Chicago field office
could not locate 5 of 17 referrals sent by a state Medicaid agency
during 1994 and 1995. As a result, it could not confirm that it

had received the referrals or explain why it had not considered
exclusion.

Our review of these five cases at the state Medicaid agency
determined that three of them involved what appeared to be serious
quality of care issues. For example, in April 1995, the Illinois
Medicaid agency excluded a dentist from its program for providing
care that placed his patients at risk of harm. Among the charges
was that the dentist had performed surgical extractions and had
given patients general anesthesia without documented need. The
state Medicaid agency's case file on this dentist showed that he
had been referred to the OIG in June 1995. When we inquired at the
Chicago field office in March 1996, however, no record could be
found of the case. Subsequent to our inquiry, the office opened a
case file on the dentist, but as of August 8, 1996, the case had
not been forwarded to headquarters for a final decision. Since
this dentist was excluded from Medicaid, he has received almost
$12,000 for services provided to Medicare patients.

When discussing weaknesses in the OIG's exclusion process with
headquarters officials, they acknowledged that improvements are
needed and informed us of a recent initiative to increase the
number and quality of exclusion cases being forwarded from the
field offices. In May 1996, the OIG began an effort to identify
all mandatory exclusion cases referred to them by the states, along
with permissive exclusion cases meeting certain criteria. Staff
performing this function will receive extra training on the
processing of provider exclusions submitted by state agencies.

OIG officials also attributed these problems to resource cuts
over the last several years. With the recent enactment of the
Health Insurance Portability and Accountability Act of 1996,
officials believe they will be able to obtain additional resources
to further address these problems.

<u>OBSERVATIONS</u>

Our work to date shows that the opportunity exists for--and
indeed we found cases in which--providers deemed to be unfit to
participate in one state's Medicaid program can continue to do so
in Medicare or in other states. Because of the amount of
communication and coordination that is needed at the state and
federal levels, the referral and exclusion process is complex.
Nevertheless, we believe that more attention must be paid to a
system that works to protect beneficiaries from substandard care
and helps ensure the integrity of federal health programs.

Although the OIG believes its initiatives and the potential
for additional investigative resources will help remedy weaknesses
in the long term, we believe that the OIG could take immediate
action in several areas that would substantially improve its
effectiveness. For example, the OIG could provide more guidance

for OIG field staff and the states to facilitate the prompt preparation of case files--including required documentation--for OIG decisions. It could also clarify guidance for the field offices to ensure more consistency in the cases that are sent forward to headquarters for a final decision. Furthermore, it could explore ways to ensure that states quickly identify and act to remove OIG-excluded providers from Medicaid participation. Finally, the OIG may want to ask states to begin reporting information on those who have agreed to withdraw from a state Medicaid program rather than subject themselves to the formal sanction process.

- - - - -

Mr. Chairman, this concludes my statement. I would be happy to respond to any questions that you or Members of the Subcommittee may have.

For more information on this testimony, please call Kathy Allen, Assistant Director, at (202) 512-7059. Other major contributors included Jon Barker, Bob Ferschl, Bob Lippencott, Al Schnupp, and Ted Wagner.

SECTIONS OF THE SOCIAL SECURITY ACT
UNDER WHICH EXCLUSIONS ARE IMPOSED

Section	Exclusion
1128(a)(1)	Program-related conviction
1128(a)(2)	Conviction for patient abuse or neglect
1128(b)(1)	Conviction related to health care fraud (non-HHS)
1128(b)(2)	Conviction related to obstruction of an investigation
1128(b)(3)	Conviction related to controlled substances
1128(b)(4)	License revocation or suspension
1128(b)(5)	Suspension or exclusion under a federal or state health care program
1128(b)(6)	Excessive claims or furnishing of unnecessary or substandard items and services
1128(b)(7)	Fraud, kickbacks, and other related activities
1128(b)(8)	Entities owned or controlled by a sanctioned individual
1128(b)(9)	Failure to disclose required information
1128(b)(10)	Failure to supply requested information on subcontractors and suppliers
1128(b)(11)	Failure to provide payment information
1128(b)(12)	Failure to grant immediate access
1128(b)(13)	Failure to take corrective action
1128(b)(14)	Default on health education loan or scholarship obligations
1128Aa	Imposition of a civil money penalty or assessment
1156(b)	Peer review organization recommendation

(101503)

Mr. SHAYS. I thank both of you for your testimony. Let me ask you, you've heard testimony from three previous witnesses. What's your general reaction to what they've told the committee? Mr. White, start with you.

Mr. WHITE. Well, I certainly have to endorse the need for a national data bank. It was talked about this morning, and I can't highlight it enough that the data that's in there has to be accessible to the States.

In New York, we have 47,000 providers who actively bill Medicaid. There are more that are enrolled in the program, but they don't actually bill, 47,000.

So in that book that you have up there, when you look at that book and we get that in to try to match it to 47,000 providers, it's a problem.

And that's what you've heard this morning.

Mr. SHAYS. It's 47,000 in your State?

Mr. WHITE. Yes.

Mr. SHAYS. Active?

Mr. WHITE. Active, actively billing the Medicaid Program. So to try to match that book to 47,000 presents obvious problems for us. So we need a data base that we can access readily.

And I'd also like to add—it wasn't talked about too much this morning—because of the process, the data base itself is not timely. It's maybe a year after the name is posted on the data base, even if it's on the Internet.

So it's not timely for us in that sense either. In fact, it presents an interesting situation where a lot of the names in that book and a lot of the actions that come back to New York are, in fact, initiated by us.

We'd throw somebody out of the Medicaid Program. We'd tell HHS. They post it a year later. Now, when we receive it today saying, "You're out for 2 years for the Federal program," we've said, "You're out for 2 years from the State program," what we end up doing is extending the exclusion for another year to match up to the Federal period of time. So that's kind of an interesting piece.

Mr. SHAYS. Why is it taking a year? I don't understand that.

Mr. WHITE. Well, I understand, from what they were saying, the State sent it to the regional office. They have to make sure——

Mr. SHAYS. OK. I'm sorry. Yes.

Dr. KOONTZ. I would reiterate what Mr. White has said. I think what happens, as far as State licensing agencies are concerned, is that we get information from the Federation State Medical Boards on a monthly basis, and we have people try to match it up.

Unfortunately, as I think Mr. Towns mentioned, something about are the State agencies all equal, and are they doing things on an equal basis as far as licensing boards, and the answer is no.

But that's why I mentioned the Federation State Medical Boards is trying to computerize it and to have electronic data transmission.

So we'll be on-line and hopefully in the next 4 to 6 months. We're just beginning to implement it now. Instead of having paper transmission, we'll be able to do that on-line.

Of course, we want to also try to keep some degree of confidentiality also, but the public information we want to get out.

Mr. SHAYS. Do both of you consider yourselves contractors for HCFA?

Mr. WHITE. In a sense.

Mr. SHAYS. Is that a comfortable thing for you to think of? I'm not trying to be coy here or cute. The bottom line is the parallel that, like with Medicare, there's 70 contractors, and you are one basic contractor for Medicaid for the Federal Government in that sense?

Mr. WHITE. In New York, I don't think we see ourselves that way, Mr. Chairman. I think we see ourselves a little more independent than that.

Mr. SHAYS. OK.

Mr. WHITE. We're concerned with the New York State Medicaid Program.

Mr. SHAYS. But ultimately, it's a lot of Federal dollars.

Mr. WHITE. Yes.

Mr. SHAYS. What I think I'm hearing you say is that you are a contractor in one sense, but you're also designing the programs and creating the programs. So you consider yourselves more than just a contractor?

Mr. WHITE. Yes.

Mr. SHAYS. OK.

Dr. KOONTZ. And the State licensing agency is different. In Virginia, for instance, we are completely separate. We get no State funds, no Federal funds. Our funds only come from fees, licensing fees and renewals.

And therefore, we're not really under contract, et cetera. We have to follow the Medical Practice Act, Drug Control Act, Administrative Process Act of the Commonwealth.

Mr. SHAYS. One of the observations that I think Mr. Souder made was that there appears to be a lot of individuals on the exclusionary list, sole practitioners or practitioners who teamed up with others.

But it seems like a lot of them are on the list. If you're a bigger operation, you probably have found a way to avoid being on that list.

Can you give us an example? A licensing board—you deal with individuals and so on.

Dr. KOONTZ. We deal with individuals.

Mr. SHAYS. Yes. But I'm just trying to get a sense of a company with a number of people that ends up ripping off the system.

Do they find a way to avoid getting that far? One of the issues is, do people get off the system before they're on the exclusionary list?

Mr. WHITE. Well, they may. What we try to do in New York, if we have any sort of corporate entity, we will try to identify the principals, the managers in that entity.

We've identified that people such as the lab medical directors, the owners of that lab, are, in fact, providers. And we will exclude them from the program as well.

So if you owned a pharmacy and we exclude the business, we will exclude you and the supervising pharmacist. So that if you try to open up another store, that will be prohibited.

Dr. KOONTZ. And with us, just to give you an anecdote, a person who has an M.D. and a Ph.D. in chemistry and wants to operate a laboratory, we can go after his M.D., but we can't do anything about his Ph.D., or his operating of the lab, because we're a licensing agency.

And if a complaint comes in about a corporation, we will go and look and see if the principals are a licensee, and then we can do something. Otherwise, we have to take it to the Commonwealth attorney, et cetera.

Mr. SHAYS. Right. But the bottom line is you can go to some other entity in the State to do that.

Dr. KOONTZ. We'd go to the Commonwealth's attorney.

Mr. SHAYS. What identifying numbers do you use for various providers of services?

Mr. WHITE. We have a State provider number that we use, if that's what you mean. Every provider in New York State has their own unique New York——

Mr. SHAYS. You have one unique number for an individual whether or not he provides different services?

Mr. WHITE. Correct. Within our Medicaid system, we identify the type of provider or the type of services that you provide.

Mr. SHAYS. But you still have one number within the State of New York?

Mr. WHITE. We have one number. We do have a backup that we use to monitor providers with. When it's a type of profession where there is a license involved, a physician, for example, we also capture the physician's license number, and we use that as a secondary means of identifying.

Mr. SHAYS. Mr. Towns.

Mr. TOWNS. Thank you very much, Mr. Chairman. Let me make certain that I clearly understand what is going on.

If a physician is excluded from the program, makes an agreement and, of course, after that's over with, he's out and then he becomes the executive director or administrator of a hospital or medical center, there is nothing you can do about that, is there?

Mr. WHITE. Well, there is really nothing we can do about it, because we probably—in most cases, we're not going to know. There are so many hospitals, that we're probably not going to know that happened.

We supply the hospitals with a list of who has been excluded, and they are required to review that and not hire people at any position within that facility.

But given the number of physicians, for example, who might be hired at a facility, it's impossible for us to tell if, in fact, everybody on that staff has been checked and cleared.

Dr. KOONTZ. I cannot tell you about Virginia Medicaid, because that's in a separate department. It's under the Department of Health. Mr. Teefey was going to be here, but he's involved with a meeting in northern Virginia. He's our Medicaid director.

But we have a mandatory statutory reporting of physicians who are either kicked off a medical staff, had their privileges restricted in any way.

So therefore, the hospital chief of staff, the hospital director have to report to us any restrictions on a physician's privileges.

Obviously, the ones that are lost are the ones who are not on any hospital staffs. You have physicians out there who are in primary care who are not on any hospital staff, belong to no organizations, and they're the ones that we're trying to get a little bit of a handle on by making them take some mandatory continued education. But that's a different problem.

Mr. TOWNS. What I'm thinking about is that you have a physician that all of a sudden is on the list or he makes an agreement and, of course, sometimes never even makes the list.

But at the same time, the way hospitals are merging, all of a sudden this person could show up as the CEO of this whole conglomerate—which means that he's now in a better position to steal or to direct others to steal than he was when he was a single practitioner out there—I don't see anything in place to deal with that situation to my satisfaction.

If I'm wrong, I would like for you to correct me, because I think fraud and abuse is a very serious issue out there.

Mr. WHITE. Well, I agree with you on that. What we have in place in New York is our regulations prohibit that from happening. That doesn't mean it doesn't happen, but that's an unacceptable practice.

Part of our regulations are directed at facilities that tell them that they are not to hire excluded providers in any capacity.

In real life, again, they could deceive us in some way. Facilities are required to submit pertinent information as part of any plan they have to consolidate or just to operate in New York.

So that information would, in fact, be available that this excluded provider is now in a management position in one of these facilities, and the regulations are in place that say this is not acceptable.

Mr. TOWNS. OK. Let me make certain that I clearly understand. And I'm really seeking information, and that's it.

Just recently, I think it was this week, in the paper, where you have a hospital from New Jersey and New York actually merging. Now, how do you control that?

So now we have a hospital in New York whose services are being provided to New York residents, but the hospital in New Jersey is also a part of this.

How do we control that? That's the question I think I'm asking. At one point we were concerned about mergers within a State, but that's no longer the problem.

Now we are merging with other hospitals in other States and all that. So I'm trying to figure out how would we get a handle on that as well.

Mr. WHITE. Well, that is a problem. You're absolutely right. A New York Medicaid recipient could receive services in that new combined facility.

Mr. TOWNS. From Connecticut or from New Jersey.

Mr. WHITE. From Connecticut or New Jersey. And it would be strictly—currently, it would be a hit and miss situation whether we knew that the New Jersey entity had, in fact, excluded providers working there.

Mr. TOWNS. And the other one I want to ask, which I would direct this to you, I'm an M.D., and have an MBA. So I use my MBA to come in to become the head of this whole medical conglomerate which you have no jurisdiction over my MBA or my master's degree in hospital administration, or whatever.

And now I come in, and I'm the same guy. The reason I'm not practicing medicine is because of the fact that I was excluded because of whatever behavior. And now I'm in charge of everything. Is there anything that can be done about that?

Dr. KOONTZ. The only thing we can do, Mr. Towns, is to refer this to the Commonwealth's attorney's office or the attorney general's office of the Commonwealth, because we only regulate the license.

And if we have withdrawn that M.D.'s license, then we cannot do anything if he or she goes into another entity and uses, as you say, his master of hospital administration, MBA, et cetera.

Then, it's going to be up to another State agency to look at them from that standpoint.

Mr. TOWNS. This is a problem, Mr. Chairman.

Dr. KOONTZ. I don't want to open another can of worms, but I know you're also, in Congress, looking at telemedicine. I mean, that's another problem with interstate medicine being practiced and how to handle that.

Mr. TOWNS. I agree. And let me say I think that New York has been very aggressive, a lot more than many of the other States in terms of trying to get a handle on this problem.

Some States are not nearly as aggressive, and I think that if we have problems in New York, then I can imagine what's happening in some of the other areas. But anyway, thank you, Mr. Chairman. I yield back.

Mr. SHAYS. I thank the gentleman. Mr. Souder. You will close up.

Mr. SOUDER. First, I don't even know for sure whether it's true, if it's not, it's a great story, and it should be true, and that is that when we first took over Congress and started redoing our computer system, supposedly hired two hackers whose job was to try to break into our systems.

And every time we broke in, then we'd plug that, because we have a lot of confidential information in our systems.

It seems to me that if not at the State level there ought to be something like this going on in the Federal level in a prioritized way.

You don't want to let anybody think that they can get away with small stuff, and pretty soon that will eat you alive.

But really, anybody who has ever watched any of the TV specials where you see the little storefronts ripping off millions of dollars or in the food stamp question where the guy up in the Baltimore stand figured out how to move $3 million through the new credit card system in, like, a week, that those type of things we ought to have—you might be, and people who run New York and some of the big States, people that say, "OK. If you were going to bust in, how would you bust into this system?"

Do you do anything like that currently in New York, or is that the job of the Federal people? Is anybody thinking in terms of, if I was going to rip this off, how would I rip you?

Mr. WHITE. Well, we don't do it from a systems perspective. We have people who work for us who are on the street.

We have Medicaid providers who cooperate with us as well, and they give us information on what's going on right now—what is the new drug on the street that people are trying to get through Medicaid to sell on the street—and that allows us to react at least fairly quickly to put some controls in on that item or whatever.

So, in a sense, we do.

Mr. SOUDER. To some degree, the media does it for you. There was the New York Post story about them being able to get people's cards and sell them and get the pills and so on.

Are there efforts by the Government to be as creative as some of the news media in discovering the fraud?

Mr. WHITE. I'd like to think so, yes. Again, like I said, we have undercover—we call them shoppers, undercover investigators who pose as Medicaid recipients who give us frontline information on what's going on, much more accurate than what the New York Post gets, I might editorialize.

Mr. SOUDER. Do you ever try to sting yourself?

Mr. WHITE. Myself?

Mr. SOUDER. Not you, but your agency, where you would set up your own front and see if you can catch it?

Mr. WHITE. Yes. We've done that.

Mr. SOUDER. I won't ask more. I don't need that. I just wanted to know if it was being done. Do you have a problem with what we heard earlier in sharing information?

In other words, if you kick somebody off your list, does that get into the feds fast?

Mr. WHITE. Yes. We send it as soon as possible to HHS–IG's regional office. What we send them is a copy of the letter that we send to providers and a copy of the summary document that we tell providers this is why we're throwing you out of the program.

So I think, in most cases, we're giving HHS some background information into what the problem is with that particular provider.

I might clarify something. I spoke how we do, on some occasions, allow providers to voluntarily withdraw in New York. I'm talking maybe a half dozen cases a year. It's not a big situation, luckily.

But in almost every single one of those instances, we've already taken steps to exclude the provider, and when we did that, we notified other insurance agencies. We notified HHS–IG.

And then somewhere down the road, because there was a problem with something going on with that case, we might have entered into this agreement.

But we've already notified people in every instance that I went back and looked at where we ended up resolving it with a voluntary——

Mr. SOUDER. Does the notification go, like, 24 hours, 2 weeks, 2 months?

Mr. WHITE. Well, they're batched. They're probably every couple weeks that we send them out.

Mr. SOUDER. I wanted to do a question also on the voluntary withdrawal. You don't mean that people can't voluntarily withdraw?

Mr. WHITE. No. They can.

Mr. SOUDER. What you mean is that once you have a pretty strong case, you don't let them voluntarily withdraw.

Mr. WHITE. We don't let you quit until we fire you.

Mr. SOUDER. We used to have a card game that was like that that had a very colorful name. If you did that, would you not just push it back, in effect, if you were a person who could see it coming?

In other words, in the start of the investigative process, do you see a higher number of people who withdraw earlier in the process, then?

Mr. WHITE. No. They can withdraw, but they withdraw in the sense that they don't bill Medicaid anymore, but that doesn't stop us from continuing our investigation of them.

Mr. SOUDER. OK.

Mr. WHITE. So they're withdrawing. Under that scenario, it has no effect whatsoever, as far as the administrative action goes.

Mr. SOUDER. I also had a couple of questions for Dr. Koontz. On your breakout of the different types of complaints that you get, if you get a fraud complaint that may relate to Medicare or Medicaid, do you just send that kind of raw to the Federal Government?

Dr. KOONTZ. We send all of our orders. I heard this morning some of the problems that they pointed out, the priority problem, and that may be something we could look at to do, because we send all of our orders to 35 different groups.

I'm sure they get deluged with a lot of paper. Some of the orders are 15, 20 pages long. So I think that's something we could improve on.

Mr. SOUDER. Do you have any idea how many of these complaints in this period actually resulted in any——

Dr. KOONTZ. About 12 percent of our complaints end up with a significant action against a licensee.

Mr. SOUDER. Do you know how many of those relate to Medicare and Medicaid?

Dr. KOONTZ. No, I don't. We have not had up to this time the electronic data to massage it to kick out that. Right now, we're using the State's mainframe downtown, and it's difficult for us to do it. We're trying to bring it all in-house in our reengineering process now.

Mr. SOUDER. Well, thank you very much for your testimony. I know it has been a long hearing.

Mr. SHAYS. It has been a long hearing, but it has been a very interesting hearing. I truly thank our third panel for their contribution.

It's not always easy to sit through the other part, but it's helpful to have your perspective, having heard those. It's interesting what your priority would be.

You come from a different perspective, and it's important to get that, and it will be included in our report.

I would like to thank our court reporter, Rita Hemphill, for her work and Tom Costa, our clerk. And also, we have an intern who has been helping us, Matthew Ebert.

And our subcommittee staff, Robert Newman has taken over for Kate Hickey, who had been handling this on a full-time basis. He has done yeoman's work. I really appreciate it, Bob. And also, our utility fielder, Cheryl Phelps, who has to be an expert on all issues, we appreciate her work.

Mr. TOWNS. You should let me say that.

Mr. SHAYS. And also has to deal with Ed Towns, which that in itself requires special recognition. With that, this hearing is adjourned.

Mr. TOWNS. I'd like to make a quick observation, though.

Mr. SHAYS. Yes.

Mr. TOWNS. I would like to just say that I noticed that Mrs. Aronovitz stayed throughout the hearing, and that, to me, I'm impressed with, because I think it points out her commitment, her dedication, because she wanted to hear not only her panel but to hear the other witnesses as well. And to me, that means a great deal.

Mr. SHAYS. I would add my second to that. I thank you for pointing that out. It's well worth pointing out. Thank you very much. This hearing is adjourned.

[Whereupon, at 1 p.m., the subcommittee was adjourned.]

○